Busting the Misinformation Harming You, Your Baby, and Society

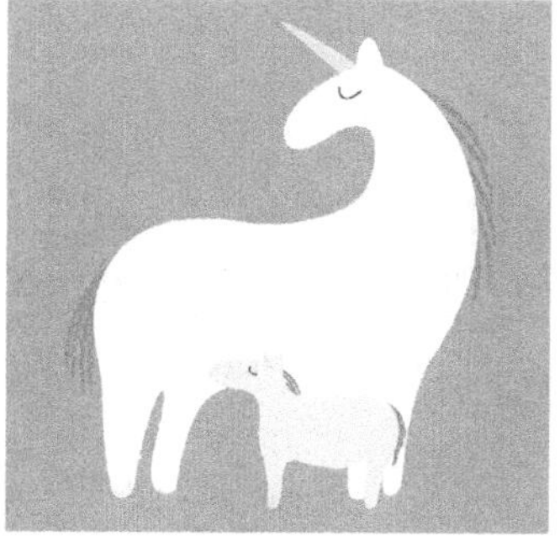

Lucy Ruddle, IBCLC

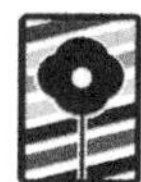

Praeclarus Press, LLC

---

www.PraeclarusPress.com

Praeclarus Press, LLC
2504 Sweetgum Lane
Amarillo, Texas 79124 USA
806-367-9950
www.PraeclarusPress.com

DISCLAIMER

The information contained in this publication is advisory only and is not intended to replace sound clinical judgment or individualized patient care. The author disclaims all warranties, whether expressed or implied, including any warranty as the quality, accuracy, safety, or suitability of this information for any particular purpose.

ISBN: 978-1-946665-55-3

Cover Design: Ken Tackett

Developmental Editing: Kathleen Kendall-Tackett

Copyediting: Chris Tackett

Layout & Design: Nelly Murariu

IMPORTANT

Throughout this book, I encourage you to seek skilled breastfeeding support. Your best options for support are, generally speaking, a national breastfeeding helpline (such as La Leche League International, the Breastfeeding Network, or National Childbirth Trust):

- A peer-support group where the volunteers have received training to help you
- A breastfeeding counsellor (again, ensure training is with a recognised national or local body for your country)
- An International Board-Certified Lactation Consultant (IBCLC)

These are the most internationally consistent ways to access support. In some parts of the world, they may be known by different names or offer slightly different training, but this is where you can find someone who is skilled in lactation support. This usually means that the person only or mostly deals with lactation. They will have some sort of specific training for breastfeeding problems, and they have sought that training that enhances their job qualifications or allows them to volunteer. Essentially, they are providing support because they want to and have gone out of their way to ensure that their training is excellent.

CONTENTS

Chapter 3

Breastfeeding Life with Your Newborn **37**

INTRODUCTION

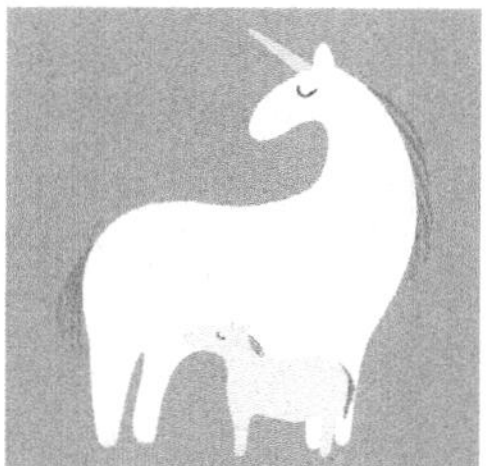

The Breastfeeding Myths That Hurt Your Chances of Success

Everyone seems to have their own opinion about breastfeeding. When you're pregnant and thinking about how you're going to feed your baby, women will tell you about how their milk never came in, how it was easy or painful, or the best thing for your baby, but you can't eat chocolate. Breastfed babies don't sleep, or breastfeeding mums get more sleep than their formula-feeding friends. The list is endless, and a lot of it is, well, nonsense. If I included every myth and random, untrue statement I've heard, this book would be too long to publish. So, I've stuck with the more common ones (and threw in a few random/odd ones, just for good measure). Where possible, I have included studies and my own clinical experience as an IBCLC to help me break down the myths that I'm discussing.

There are thick, academic tomes in human lactation. We don't need another one, so I've kept the tone light and readable. When we're talking about some absurd myth I use humour to avoid crying.

There are also some more serious topics because, sadly, more than a few myths have hurt breastfeeding families. Breastfeeding can be an emotional topic. Take care of yourself while reading and skip anything that upsets you, or feels too big or close to home.

I've written this book for you to flick through or read from start to finish. It's in a logical order: —societal issues, antenatal, newborns, older babies, toddlers, etc.—but each myth is short and clearly headed so you can skip to the bits you need.

For the most part, I hope this book finds its way to somewhere it can be picked up and read for a bit of entertainment, as well as education. I won't be offended if that happens in your bathroom. Enjoy!

CHAPTER 1

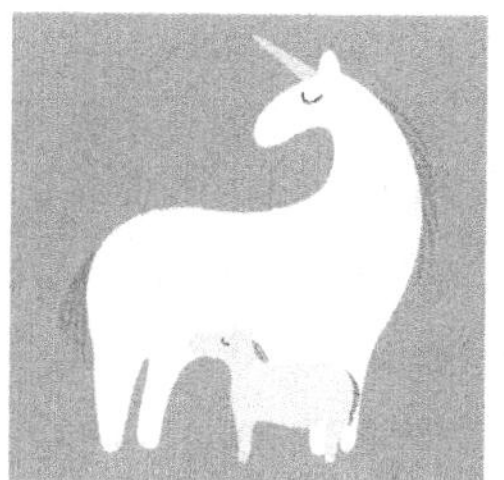

How and Why a Formula-Feeding Society Spreads Misinformation

Many people find this topic difficult. It's hard to think about the underhanded methods formula companies use without looking like I am judging people who use or have used formula. They don't believe that formula is the norm in the West because they felt pressured to breastfeed.

When I say that formula is seen as normalised, I mean that formula is often offered as the solution to any breastfeeding problem. If you live in the UK, most of your peers started using formula by the time their babies are 6 weeks old. Pictures of bottles show you where baby-care rooms are in supermarkets, shopping centres, and airports. On daytime TV, social media, and local radio, people still debate about whether breastfeeding in public should be allowed, even though the law in the UK protects your right to feed your baby anywhere you can be. This is what a formula-feeding society looks like.

A Short History

You were born into a formula-using culture. You were probably formula-fed (at least in part). You may have heard horror stories about breastfeeding, or even experienced it first-hand. How did formula get to be so influential? More than 100 years ago, formula worked its way into society. Let's start with the society-wide issue that this normalisation brings.

"Mothers will do my publicity for me," said Henri Nestle about his formula milk back in the 1800s. Even today, they still use parents to promote formula products. Ask most people which formula they think you should use, and they will probably claim that the brand their baby took is best. Unless they still remember the quickly banned advert from a particular UK formula brand that claimed their product was the closest to breastmilk. It's not just parents. Formula companies send you glossy leaflets or pregnancy diaries when you signed up for their baby club. This is nothing more than marketing tactics. Their helplines are an extension of this and are as close to milk nurses as they can get.

What are milk nurses? Formula companies, predominantly Nestle, hired women to dress as nurses and distribute formula to mothers and healthcare providers, typically in developing countries, saying that it was better than mothers' milk. Their title of "milk *nurse*" meant that many parents, especially poor mothers in the developing world, thought they were healthcare providers and that they were there to help them to feed their babies. Unfortunately, their jobs were simply to sell Nestle-branded formula.

These "nurses" would use tactics, like one described in the 1974 article, "The Baby Killer" by Mike Muller. Muller describes how an uninvited milk nurse approached a mother living in a developing country in her home. This "nurse" explained that if the mother intended to breastfeed, she would need to give the baby a fairly long list of extra vitamins, juices, and supplements, but if she used a formula milk, this would cut out the need for these added extras. Just imagine having a new baby, worrying about all sorts of things, and then someone in a nurse's uniform knocks on your door and tells you that giving your baby formula will be easier. You get a free tin of formula to get you started and then stop breastfeeding as a result. Then you must find the money for the powder every week. You need a clean source of water, the ability to heat it, and a way to clean your equipment. Imagine later finding out that your breastmilk already contained *all* the "extras" you thought you needed to buy and prepare separately if you wanted to breastfeed.

History of Formula

We can't go any further into this book without a bit of background information about formula milk. The commercialisation of formula was a dangerous and unprecedented tipping point for breastfeeding around the world. That said, please know that I'm *not* against the use of formula: many, many of the parents I support use it, and my last book was about how to use formula alongside human milk. What I am against, however, is the formula *industry* and its money-above-health attitude towards mothers and babies the world over.

We need to understand, of course, that people have wanted an alternative to breastmilk for much of human history. Wet nursing has a long history. Babies who weren't wet-nursed or fed at their own mother's breast were given animal milk alongside a range of other inappropriate foods. This contributed to the deaths of countless infants.

In some ways, the advent of formula was something to celebrate. It saved lives and still does. Sadly, it also claimed many lives due to its inadequate nutritional make up, being used where it isn't needed, or when it was undermined by poor hygiene practices. In fact, despite considerable improvements to both the milk and the way we are taught to prepare it, formula still can lead to infant mortality where it isn't used appropriately or safely. For example, a 2018 study found that the availability of formula increased infant mortality by 9.4 per 1,000 births (95% CI [confidence interval]) where clean water was difficult to access (Anttila-Hughes et al., 2018).

Formula was initially complicated. Parents were told to skim off the fat from cows' milk and add sugar and lime water (lime water being calcium hydroxide) in order to make milk for their babies to drink. This would be difficult for tired new mothers to manage.

It was only a matter of time before an easily soluble "complete infant food" became popular. Henri Nestle and Baron von Liebig extensively promoted these types of formula to mothers and the medical community. These milks claimed to be a perfect substitute for mother's milk, even though they lacked some essential ingredients. So, despite these somewhat improved milks, babies were still dying from lack of human milk. There are many upsetting stories of babies failing to thrive until a wet nurse was employed. However, by the middle of the 20th century, most babies were fed formula milk. By this point, most considered it to be safe, thanks to steps taken to understand how to make a nutritionally complete milk for human babies and how to ensure that milk is safely prepared and stored.

Today's infant formula is nutritionally complete but still lacks many of the ingredients you will find in breastmilk. This includes stem cells and antibodies that provide significant protection for the baby's developing immune system. Formula has a place in supporting babies' growth when breastmilk is not available. Unfortunately, formula marketing practices are often so damaging that many infants receive formula as their main source of nutrition unnecessarily and against the desires of their parents. More importantly, many mothers are not reaching their personal breastfeeding goals because society was in the pocket of an unethically run formula industry; an industry that puts profits above the health of our most vulnerable members of society.

Parenting Practices and Formula Vs. Breast

We live in a world where a good baby sleeps all night, feeds every four hours, and is then happy to kick his legs on a play mat for an hour while his caregiver (usually Mum) cleans the house, exercises, and prepares a healthy family dinner. These expectations became noticeable when formula-feeding became the norm and coincided with when women worked outside the home on a more regular basis. Breastfeeding was time-consuming and problematic when you had to work several hours a day. However, if your baby could be given a big bottle of milk and then be content for several hours, then that was one less thing to worry about.

Around the same time, it became normal for us to manipulate baby feeding and sleep patterns, even when we had better breastfeeding initiation rates and better maternity leave. We have gotten used to how babies with bellies overfull of formula behave, and are less used to how exclusively breastfed babies behave. Normal breastfeeding behaviours become problems to be solved, with the often-overfed bottle baby being seen as normal. Still, many parents and professionals today believe that babies should be fed every 3 or 4 hours, and should be sleeping 10 to 12 hours at night. Even adults do not do this. Why do we expect that babies who can't scratch an itch, take themselves to the toilet, grab a sip of water, or soothe themselves back to sleep can?

Breast Is Best/Fed Is Best

People often think that these statements are lovely, warm, and inclusive. Unfortunately, they have only served to divide us. Do you know what I think is best? Individual support that provides evidence-based information given with empathy and no judgement. I guess that isn't as divisive, catchy, or cheap to provide.

Where do these terms come from? Breast is Best is a phrase possibly created by a formula company somewhere. Why would they want to use that phrase? To make breastfeeding seem like something only the best people can do. Think of other things that fall into "the best" category: eating your five servings a day of fruit and vegetables, getting an Oxbridge education, exercising for 30 minutes five times a week, sleeping for eight hours every night, avoiding sugar; things that are hard to achieve perfectly. If something is "best," it's probably hard to do. Formula provides the other the thing that most people can achieve.

> *During pregnancy I was always told "breast is best." A leaflet in my red book highlighted this and had some stats on how formula increases the risks of many things, such as SIDS, leukaemia, etc., so I was then beside myself on day 5, when we were readmitted to hospital for 13.9% weight loss and I needed formula, as I couldn't pump enough for the top ups she needed.* ◆ **Katie**

If formula is seen as second best, then it's *almost* the best, right? It's second. Second is good. You'd be proud to come second in a competition (as long as you didn't lose out on a million-pound prize). So, if we try to make formula seem *second best*, then it must be a *good* thing.

Except "second best," according to the World Health Organisation, would be Mum's milk pumped. If that's not available, then third best is someone else's milk. WHO considers formula to be fourth best for babies.

There's that word again: best. Yet, feeding your baby cannot be broken down to "best" or "second best" categories. You've got a whole new human there, who is going to grow up to live their life, with challenges and successes. Surely, they just need food as a baby, and it doesn't matter what that food is, as long as Mum doesn't feel guilty for the sort of milk being fed? Is it a case of Fed is Best?

No.

All babies must be fed. It's not a choice. "Oh well, it's best if you feed your baby, but you know... probably okay if you don't" would be a statement worthy of someone losing their entire healthcare career.

The term Fed is Best silences parents who are upset about using formula, and it may be that we don't know how to help and want to make ourselves feel more comfortable. "Don't worry about it; fed is best, after all!" Those words are usually shared with love and kindness at their core. We don't want someone to be upset about stopping breastfeeding; we want to take away that pain and help them to see what an amazing parent they are. Breastfeeding grief is powerful, painful stuff that doesn't disappear when everyone has moved on to other topics. Breastfeeding grief can last for *years*. Do you know how we heal grief and trauma like this? We feel our feelings and we talk about them. We don't swallow them because we feel silly, thanks to everyone banging on about fed is best. Several generations carry that grief. They were told that fed is best instead of being offered actual breastfeeding support. Instead of silencing mothers, we should let them talk. Plenty of evidence suggests that talking about difficult experiences helps humans to heal and find acceptance, rather than carrying those feelings for decades to come (Ford et al., 2018).

I was told "fed is best" on many occasions. Although I know most people mean well, to me, every time I heard that phrase, it just screamed, "I'm not considering your feelings here, Mumma." It really hurt me and made me feel like all my efforts weren't valid or good enough, and that I didn't have my baby's best interests at heart, therefore, making me feel like a bad mum. ◆ **Gemma**

So, no, fed is not best but neither can we say breast is best. Supported, informed, and empowered; those things are best for all families.

Sexualisation of Breasts

Remember the Wonder Bra billboards that reportedly had men crashing their cars? Yeah, that's one reason we have a big problem with breastfeeding in the West. Not because of Eva Herzigova's breasts, as such, but because of the way we, as a society, have made breasts to be so distracting and exciting for men that they are at risk of smashing up their vehicles when faced with a giant pair of boobs. There are societies in this world where, if you told the men we sexualise breasts in the West, you would be laughed at and called a baby. In their culture, breasts are for feeding children, not for men to ogle over. I remember being told that on the islands of Laos in the 1800s, unmarried women and children covered their breasts, but once married, they would stop doing this and have their breasts exposed, as they needed them to feed babies and children.

Yes, I know nipples are sensitive to stimulation and it can feel good to have them touched in a sexual relationship. However, hands, necks, lips, and ears are all also erogenous zones, and no one is demanding we cover those up. Some people are into feet, too, yet we can still walk barefoot on the beach without being told to put socks on because some guy over there finds feet sexy and doesn't think the beach is an appropriate place to have them on display.

Once, this older woman came over to me while I was feeding, and she told me I needed to cover up because her husband was embarrassed to see me with my breasts exposed! Luckily for me, I was in a breastfeeding-friendly café and the manager invited the couple to move or leave. ◆ **Liz**

I live by the beach and every summer I swear I see men with bigger boobs than some of the mums I support. All uncovered, no problems at all, yet taking sideways glances at the female breasts covered in material nearby. It reminds me of the game you can play where you're shown breast tissue with no context, and you have to guess if it's male or female. The *only* reason female breast tissue is sexualised is because it is found on the female body.

The primary function of breasts is to feed babies. Mammals have breast tissue that secretes milk. Ever see someone asking a chimp, a cow, or a sheep to cover up their mammary glands because it's inappropriate to be feeding her young in public? No, me neither.

So, the myth that breasts are just for sex? No truer than our hands and mouths being for sex.

Profits Above Health

People assume that the government and the companies who sell us baby products want to help us to look after babies. After all, who doesn't want to protect babies? Unfortunately, the answer to that is anyone with a financial interest in babies not being breastfed, and a government that neither knows nor cares about the importance of breastmilk for reducing long-term costs elsewhere. Money speaks, and sadly for us, lactation is free. (At least in the traditional sense of the word, there is a lot to be said about the value of women's time and work in raising babies, but that is probably for a different book.)

Formula companies are particularly clever at looking as though they care about parents and babies, from their glossy ads with carefully chosen slogans to their helplines staffed by midwives and other professionals. They give away teddies, vouchers, and send you monthly emails about your baby's development. They're so generous! Except, if you formula-feed, you're paying for these things. The £10 you pay for a tin of formula is not what it costs to produce; the markup is huge.

Yes, companies should be able to make a profit on their products, but, ideally, essential food for babies should never have been a commercial product. Formula is supposed to be a medical aid to support the growth of infants who don't have access to breastmilk. Medical aids in the UK are usually provided freely, or cheaply, through the NHS. If formula was treated as the lifesaving medicine it truly is, then you wouldn't have to pay £10-12 a tin and be told every 2 minutes that you need to "move on" from breastfeeding and give your baby follow-on milk. The NHS would have more incentive to support people who want to breastfeed, and no one would have to water down their baby's formula because they can't afford the stuff.

Some people reading this will say, "that's not fair. You shouldn't have to get past a doctor to give your baby formula." I doubt this would be the issue we anticipate. They give Gaviscon to children like it's water. In Scotland, Gaviscon prescriptions for infants increased from 15% to 24% between 2010 and 2016 (Cowie, Holland, Pirie, & Milliagan 2016). No doctor worth their salt would refuse to prescribe the thing babies need to stay alive. It *would* mean you would have an opportunity to talk about why you want to stop breastfeeding/not breastfeed in the first place, though. If formula being on prescription means that the government steps up their funding for breastfeeding support to save money, then you might even get a better chance of seeing an actual breastfeeding specialist on the NHS to help you overcome your problems.

In short, formula companies make a lot of money from when people formula-feed. They are more interested in your money than in your baby's health and describe breastfeeding as "a problem" to deal with so they can sell more milk. Formula companies push their prices up to promote it more, so they stop more people breastfeeding, not because the product is particularly difficult or expensive to make. Formula companies directly damage the goals of those wanting to breastfeed *and* make formula unnecessarily expensive for those who need or choose to use it.

> *If you have never struggled to keep your family fed, you won't understand the guilt from having to water down formula. I only did it twice,*

but both times, I was so scared she would get sick as a result. I had no help breastfeeding and no money to pay for formula as well as keeping my older child fed . . . it's honestly disgusting that this can happen in 21st century Britain. ◆ **Anonymous**

In 2010, I gave birth to my eldest son. I was a 20-year-old, newly divorced, first-time mother. I had left my job before my son's birth, so I was navigating the complicated benefits system, which resulted in months of no government assistance. I was receiving £50 per week income support, which would have to cover food, bills, clothes, formula, etc.

I intended to breastfeed but had very little professional support and my immediate family pressured me into formula-feeding. I combi-fed for as long as possible but eventually, my son was completely formula-fed.

There were many times I didn't eat so I would have enough money for formula. I never watered his formula down because I knew about the potential health risks. As a young mother, I was so scared to reach out for help, as I thought social services may intervene and potentially take my son away. I felt like such a failure.

Looking back, I wish I had easy access to things like food banks, etc. and that it was easier to ask for help without the stigma or fear. ◆ **Sinead**

Medical Training

How much training do you think a GP has had in lactation? Maybe a series of lectures at university? An assignment? Some supervised experience in a breastfeeding setting? We assume that doctors and paediatricians are experts because breastfeeding is covered in their training, right? Sadly not. Most doctors, nurses, and paediatricians have little to no breastfeeding education. If they do, it is about one lecture. Maybe. Possibly funded and delivered by a formula company. The same is true for nursing education.

The only education we had on lactation was a group presentation where we chose to look at breastmilk vs. formula ingredients for the topic. We got backlash from others in our class because they had a hard time breastfeeding. ◆ **A nurse.**

Thankfully, there is a movement to improve this. The GP Infant Feeding Network, as well as the Hospital Infant Feeding Network (both UK-based), are working hard to get better breastfeeding knowledge into the medical world. But, as of now, chances are that if you go to your doctor with a breastfeeding problem, you will come away with one of three (usually unnecessary) things following a ten-minute consultation:

1. A prescription for reflux medication
2. A prescription for thrush treatment
3. Instructions to stop breastfeeding

You might get all three, and a prescription for antidepressants. The biggest problem is that because these people have a lot of education, we believe that they are correct. In contrast, if you presented to an IBCLC with painful breastfeeding and a fussy, apparently refluxy baby, they would:

1. Gather a full history about you and your baby
2. Examine your breasts
3. Examine your baby's mouth
4. Observe a breastfeed and help you to reduce your pain
5. Explain how improving latching or adjusting milk flow can help with fussing/funny coloured nappies/vomiting
6. Talk with you about biologically normal infant behaviour (i.e., not wanting to be put down, appearing to be uncomfortable, and not sleeping much unless held)

Other breastfeeding-trained supporters would do the same.

In other words, if you see a breastfeeding supporter, they will figure out what's going on and help you to continue to breastfeed. Yes, if they think you actually have thrush or a refluxy baby, they will suggest you see the doctor too.

There's a deeper issue at play here as well. A lot of people looking after new parents may have had their own negative experiences of breastfeeding, where personal experience trumps evidence-based practice. Take my own GP as an example: "You've done 2 weeks and really it's not that important to carry on. I was formula-fed and I'm a doctor! My children were formula-fed and they are the fittest men you could meet!"

Sadly, it's not the doctors' fault they had no training or experience needed to effectively support parents with lactation and infant feeding issues. The problem is, once again, lack of funding, lack of understanding, and a general lack of care from society at large when it comes to feeding babies.

> *Everything I learned about breastfeeding, I learnt from being a mother.*
>
> ◆ **A paediatrician**

Medical professionals (whether doctors, nurses, or midwives) don't get to debrief on their own feeding experiences when they return from maternity leave. Medical professionals told me while writing this section that they dreaded breastfeeding coming up with their patients because it hurt too much to talk about, even in a clinical way. These people are meant to offer support, but they weren't supported themselves. As a comparison, most lactation-specific training, whether voluntary or professional, asks you to talk and/or write about your own breastfeeding experience at least once before you qualify. I had multiple debriefs at each stage of my training.

If medical professionals are not guaranteed to be able to support you with your breastfeeding problems or worries, where can you turn?

In the UK, midwives know more than doctors about breastfeeding. Midwives undergo lactation training as part of their qualifications, although this isn't as in-depth as you might imagine. A Breastfeeding Counsellor has had more training than your average midwife. Having said this, the midwifery team can usually get you off to a good start with feeding, if they have the time to do so. The biggest issue in UK maternity units is that everyone is so overworked and time-poor that, despite some real feeding experts being available, you just might not get access to the right person on the right day.

Peer Support Groups

The UK has some great free resources where you can get breastfeeding support. There are peer support groups where breastfeeding mums volunteer to support other parents in their community. These volunteers have some good basic training in breastfeeding support and are good listeners.

National Helplines

There are different helplines to offer breastfeeding support in the UK and around the world. These are generally run by volunteers who have had about 18 months to 2 years of breastfeeding and counselling training.

The Drugs in Breastmilk Information Service

Run by pharmacists, this excellent source is where parents and medical professionals turn to when a question comes up about drugs and breastfeeding. The InfantRisk Center is a similar organization in the U.S.

Your Local Infant Feeding Team

Typically made up of hospital support workers, your local infant feeding team is trained in breastfeeding support and can often see you at home, even after you've been discharged by midwifery. This isn't always the case, though, as it depends on your individual hospital's service.

Of course, you should seek medical advice if you are experiencing problems. The purpose of this chapter is not to convince you to avoid it. However, if a doctor or similar person tells you to stop breastfeeding and use formula (against your better judgement), or tells you that you can't take certain medication while breastfeeding, check with breastfeeding support organisations to make sure you've got all the information available. You need information to make an informed choice.

> *We had two lectures on breastfeeding in 4 years at medical school, which focused on benefits to the child and the mother, WHO recommendations, a bit about mastitis and blocked ducts, and came with cautionary discussions about safe medications to prescribe in breastfeeding mums.*

> *Not once did any lecture talk about troubleshooting issues with latch, express feeding, combi-feeding, or the things that would be helpful for supporting a mum who wants to feed but is struggling. I'd love more education for GPs like me.* ◆ **A GP**

I'd like to take a moment to acknowledge the hard work so many healthcare providers are undertaking to improve this situation for their colleagues and the families they support. Thank you for shifting the narrative of an entire country.

I've decided to conclude this chapter with the following description from Rachel. She submitted her story for my section on tongue-tie. However, what she demonstrates so well with her experience is an unintentional lack of appropriate care from the medical professionals around her, leading to her baby being tube fed when it's likely this shouldn't have needed to happen if training, staffing levels, and funding were up to scratch.

> In hospital, baby aged 8 weeks and constantly distressed, me equally distressed and exhausted. Baby had been on feeding plans since birth, nipple shields, and top ups. Readmitted for failure to gain weight.
>
> Nurse: "We think you have an oversupply so you're not giving him the fatty milk. Here's a pump; express before you feed him, so you remove the fore-milk."
>
> Me: "I think the problem is still his tongue-tie. He struggles to latch onto a bottle for his top ups and cannot naturally latch to the breast. I don't think he is transferring milk as well as he could be" reiterated this to every nurse and every doctor.
>
> Doctor: "There doesn't seem to be a problem with his tongue, let's try this pumping out for 24 hours and see what happens." The second paediatrician to "investigate" said that there is no issue. By this point, he's had a procedure done twice already.
>
> Oh, and I had to do this on my own, juggling pumping, washing, sterilising, explosive nappies, with the baby crying almost constantly (Note: Everyone was kind, but COVID didn't help).

Me: Despairingly agreed to the pumping before a feed. Then, continuing the bottle top ups.

After two sessions of doing this:

Me: Running out of clothing and muslins for us both. "This isn't working; he just brings it all back up again."

Middle of the night: The baby is lethargic and I'm increasingly worried, as are the staff.

Nurse: "Okay, I've spoken to the doctors. Are you happy for us to pop in an NGT? Or try formula?"

Me: Exhausted and worried about my little boy, "Yes, okay, let's try the NGT with BM."

Next 24hrs: Breastfed and NGT BM at the same time.

Meanwhile...

Thinks he has CMPA. Discussed options and they agreed to breastfeed and remove allergens from my diet and top up with Neocate. At this point, I'm so worried about him, that the formula input was less of an issue.

Weight gain attributed to the Neocate. NGT out.

Another day or so being covered in sick, omeprazole increased to weight limit, stable enough to leave hospital for the night and back to check the following day. Did so, all stable. Review in a few weeks.

Neocate: Bought up after every feed along with the breastmilk. Told them I'd go back to BM top ups.

Breastfeeding: Still long, long feeds, poor latch.

Weight: Falling and ended up at below the 2nd.

Made the decision to have his tongue-tie looked at privately at 15 weeks.

Tongue-tie still present! Surprise, surprise! Had the procedure done and some IBCLC breastfeeding support, as well as continuing input from a cranial osteopath. Dropped top ups.

Baby has thrived since, up, up, up on the growth charts and is now between the 50th and 75th. Feeds now under 10 mins, happy content baby, less sickness.

Subsequent review appointments. Doctor pleased with gains but no acknowledgement that I was in fact right all along, with the fact it was his tongue-tie (although I don't dispute the CMPA having an impact).

One happy baby boy, one happy mummy! We still have some problems, allergies, oral damage, so weaning is a challenge and awaiting oral surgery. Omeprazole still needed, now lactulose for constipation. However, he's breastfeeding! He's thriving and enjoying exploring the world around him, and finally, we are properly able to enjoy him!

CHAPTER 2

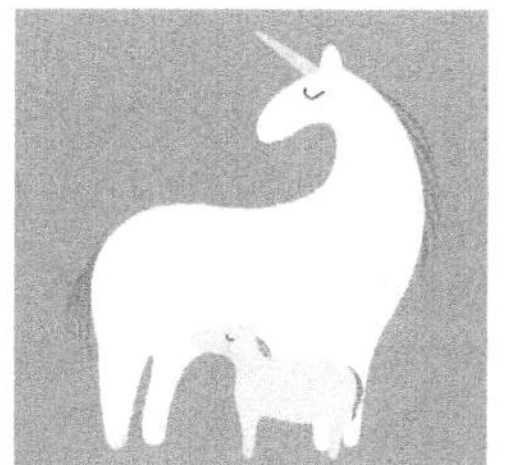

Things You're Told Before Your Baby Is Born

You get to enjoy some weird and wonderful nonsense about lactation while you're pregnant. A lot of the misinformation is well intentioned. Or people may simply share their experiences and stories with you. They can range from scary to odd. Keep in mind that you will encounter people from multiple generations who formula-fed. It's not surprising that your great aunt or mother-in-law have some horror stories to share because they likely had little support or correct information when they had their own babies.

Most of the myths I describe in this chapter plant big seeds of doubt in your mind but squashing them with some science and experience should help you to regain your confidence in your body and baby.

Formula Is So Good These Days, That It's Not Much Different to Breastmilk

At its core, formula is cows' milk (or soy) that is processed to make it suitable for human babies who have access to clean water. It grows babies well, and has an important place where breastmilk isn't an option or wanted. However, breastmilk has millions of live cells in it, as well as over 1,000 proteins and 200 complex sugars that feed the good bacteria in the baby's gut (Ballard & Morrow, 2013). There are also growth factors and hormones that do things like help regulate appetite and sleep patterns. There are also five different types of antibodies in human milk, and their job is to help protect babies against illnesses. Therefore, breastfed babies are less likely to get sick, and if they do, they tend to get better faster than their formula-fed peers. On a similar note, there are 1,400 micoRNAs in your milk. These help to stop diseases progressing and even remodel the breast (Alsaweed et al., 2016).

People can get upset when we talk about the amazing ingredients in breastmilk compared to formula, which is a shame. If we can step back from the feelings and think about it, we realize how incredible it is that female bodies can make this amazing thing like it's no big deal.

Low Supply Is Common

Some myths blossom from a grain of truth. Low milk supply is a great example of that. Low supply is fairly common in the West, but this isn't because we don't make milk well. It's because several things tend to happen in the first few weeks that cause it, like:

- Ineffective feeding (and you're usually told the feeding is totally fine).
- Missed feedings (deliberately spaced feeding, or unintentional causes, such as a difficult-to-wake baby).
- Limited support protecting milk supply if your baby needs formula or donor milk top-ups.

These issues reduce milk removal. Reduced milk removal lowers milk supply because if milk is not removed, your body thinks the milk isn't needed and it slows down milk production.

Of course, a percentage of women *do* experience physiological low milk supply (sometimes called primary low milk supply), and this will be caused by something being a bit out of kilter with Mum's breasts or hormones. Primary low milk supply is fairly rare, and low supply doesn't mean no supply. It also doesn't mean your baby can't breastfeed. For some people, it may mean the baby needs to have formula or donor milk, as well as Mum's own milk. Primary low milk supply is triggered by issues such as:

- Retained placenta
- Limited breast tissue
- Thyroid dysfunction
- PCOS (in some cases)
- Breast surgery (in some cases)

My top tips for parents worried about low milk supply would be to make sure feeding is totally and completely spot on, and if you're having feeding challenges to make sure you're expressing milk to maintain a milk supply while working things out.

> I have very obvious hypoplastic breasts. No one thought to tell me this might be the cause of my low supply! It took nine weeks and two IBCLCs to have someone suggest [that] maybe I really did have primary low supply.

If you think your low supply is caused by something physical, it can be helpful to remember that the power of breastmilk is dose responsive: the more we give, the better the outcome. *Any* amount supports your baby's immune system. One recent study found that any breastmilk feeding reduced a baby's risk of sudden infant death syndrome; the more the baby breastfed, the lower the risk (Thompson et al., 2017).

Your Breasts Are Too Small to Produce Milk

If you're thirsty, you fetch yourself a glass of water. If you are pouring your water into a pint glass, you will only need to fill it once. If you use a shot glass, you will need to refill it many times to satisfy your thirst. The tap still produces all the water you need. Your breasts are like the shot glass/pint glass, and your body is like the tap. It will make milk as long as your baby removes that milk. You might have what we call a small storage capacity (shot-glass boobs), so your baby might want to feed more often. Interestingly, milk storage capacity has little to do with breast size.

What is milk storage capacity? It's the amount of milk your breasts can hold when they are at their fullest. As I discuss above, this is different for every single person. Mohrbacher (2010) explains that some mums have a storage capacity of 2.6 oz., while others can hold 20.5 oz, with every amount in between. Your milk-making tissue determines your storage capacity, not your size.

Most babies take around 750-900ml of milk per day. If you have a small storage capacity, your baby might want to feed from both breasts and feed often. If you have a large storage capacity, they might only want to feed from one breast and be happy going for three hours or more without feeding. Fortunately, Kent et al. (2006) found that babies whose mums had a low milk storage capacity still gained weight well when they were fed responsively.

So, do small boobs mean you can't make enough milk? No. Smaller breasts might have a smaller storage capacity than bigger breasts, but that's not always the case. If it is, your baby can just feed more often.

> *I breastfed my little boy for just over 3 years with breasts that I would say are small, a handful is what I would call my breasts. Throughout our 3-year journey, I never had an issue with supply. It never entered my head that breast size would effect milk supply and thankfully, I had a brilliant local support group who helped me understand that breast size did not affect milk supply. It was the way I responded to my little boy's needs for milk that kept my supply going.* ◆ **Becks**

> *I'm a small B-cup. I breastfed my little girl for over 3 years. I never once thought that because I had small breasts, I'd fail to feed. I just fed my baby on demand whenever she wanted it and that helped my supply.* ◆ **Sasha**

You Have Flat or Inverted Nipples So You Won't Be Able to Breastfeed

While a flat or inverted nipple can make breastfeeding harder, the way your nipples are in pregnancy doesn't tell us anything useful. Hormones often draw the nipple out as pregnancy progresses, and especially when the oxytocin hits after birth. We also can't be sure that an inverted nipple will stay that way once baby is feeding. Often, the baby can draw them out well. The average nipple gets to double its usual length during feedings.

If flat or inverted nipples make breastfeeding harder for your baby, there are ways around this.

- You could draw your nipple out with an evertor, breast pump, or your fingers before feeding.
- You could use a nipple shield.

We used to recommend using breast shells, and other devices, in pregnancy to help pull nipples into an erect position ready for the baby's birth. However, more recent research has found these to be ineffective.

One fact I especially like is that nipples tend to become less inverted the longer you breastfeed and with each subsequent lactation. So, nipples that start off hidden with your first baby will probably be pointy and ready for action by baby number two or three.

Nipple Shields Will Reduce Your Milk Supply and Stop Your Baby from Breastfeeding Well

Nipple shields get such a bad reputation, but they have saved many a breastfeeding relationship when used correctly in the right situation. Handing out nipple shields to postnatal parents like sweets is not a good idea because we do want to support babies feeding without them. Some concerns regarding shields include that they can reduce milk removal and they can encourage a poor latch because you won't feel as much pain.

Having said that, nipple shields can be used effectively (with trained support) for a few reasons, including:

- A premature baby
- A baby with a high palate
- Relactation
- Induced lactation (where your baby hasn't been breastfed before)
- Flat or inverted nipples
- To allow damage to heal if you are also correcting the underlying cause of that damage

So, while not the first step, nipple shields certainly are not the problem they are often assumed to be.

> *(I was told) using breast shields will cause nipple confusion. I struggled to get started with breastfeeding, my boobs were just so engorged, my baby couldn't get a good latch. My sister went and got me some nipple shields in the hope they would help extend my nipple reach, so to speak, and it worked. After a week, my engorgement settled down, and I was able to stop using the shields.* ◆ **Susannah**

It Will Hurt

The idea that breastfeeding should/will hurt is pervasive in our Western world. Ask a group of parents if feeding their baby was painful and most, if not all, will say "yes." Over the last few years, I have heard the following (untrue) reasons about why breastfeeding hurts:

- The nipples need to toughen up
- It's because the mother has red hair

- It's because the parent has white skin
- It's because the mother has freckles
- Pain means that it's working
- There's no cause for the pain
- It's just that the parent has a low pain threshold

Within the first couple of days of having my first baby, I was told by a midwife that my nipple pain might be because "redheads have sensitive skin." Spoiler: That wasn't the issue! ◆ **Hannah**

The trouble is that breastfeeding isn't supposed to hurt. So, if all of the above is not true, why does breastfeeding hurt so often in the early days? Generally, it's down to positioning and attachment being poor or not quite right. This includes:

- Tongue-tie
- Large nipples and a small baby
- A high palate
- The parent and baby needing time to find the best way to fit together
- A sleepy newborn
- A crying newborn

We had "slight" tongue-tie, which the hospital said wouldn't cause issues. It did! ◆ **Donna**

Why do these positioning and attachment issues lead to pain? Inside your baby's mouth is a hard palate (at the front) and a soft palate (near the back); the hard palate is bony, and the soft palate is cushiony. Where would you like your nipple to be resting? The soft palate, obviously. However, because it's so far back in the baby's mouth, it can be tricky to get your nipple far enough back in the early days. This is especially so if your baby is too sleepy to open their mouth wide or screaming too much to get their tongue down and out of the way. Instead, we end up with your nipple being compressed between your baby's tongue (or lower gum, if you're unlucky) and the hard palate at the front of their mouth. That's going to hurt. It's also going to cause nipples that are:

- Blanched
- Squashed
- Pinched
- Flattened on one side
- Blistered
- Cracked
- Bleeding
- Inflamed

As well as causing a mum to wonder how she can possibly keep going through this much pain. If breastfeeding hurts, something needs adjusting. Pain tells your body that something is wrong, and if breastfeeding was supposed to be painful, we would have died out millennia ago. Also, consider every other mammal; no dog or chimpanzee would tolerate painful lactation. They'd move away from their young if it hurt to feed them. Feeding our young is supposed to be comfortable because our survival depended on it. If you don't put up with a shoe rubbing against your little toe, the wrong prescription of glasses, a bra that is too tight, or the way a pretty headband can give you those debilitating headaches of death (or is that just me?), then don't put up with a painful latch.

So now that we are clear that breastfeeding shouldn't hurt, what can you do if it does? First, ignore anyone who tells you there is no reason for your pain, and instead, find someone who is better qualified to be assessing infant-feeding issues. That may well be another midwife, an infant feeding support worker, a maternity assistant, a particular health visitor, a peer supporter, a breastfeeding counsellor, or an IBCLC.

There are so many ways you can access support; you just need to know how and where to do so.

> *I was told repeatedly that my latch was fine and that my son was feeding well. Breastfeeding became extremely painful (this was misdiagnosed as thrush), and my son hardly gained any weight for 2 months. Eventually, I saw a private IBCLC who addressed poor positioning and shallow latch, and we managed to get back on track, but being fobbed off and in constant pain for weeks was incredibly damaging to my mental health. I felt absolutely useless and like I was letting my son down not being able to get help.* ◆ **Lyndsay**

There are some basics you can try while waiting to get in-person support.

1. Make sure you are comfy. Leaning back slightly actually helps more than sitting upright for most mums, as gravity can help to "smush" the baby in close to your body.

2. Try to be skin-to-skin with your baby if you can. Skin-to-skin makes the most of feeding reflexes and ensures that no clothes get in the way of the baby or breast. At the very least, have your baby's cheek on your breast.

3. Turn your baby so their tummy and chest are touching your front. This seems to help babies feel safe and grounded, ready for feeding, as well as making sure that they don't have to stretch too far to get the breast.

4. Have your baby lined up so the tip of their nose (above the nostrils) is touching your nipple. (I know it feels counterintuitive, but they *should* tip their heads back in this position, sending the nipple far back to the soft palate.)

5. When your baby gapes, push them in towards you firmly and quickly by the shoulders. Do *not* move your nipple to your baby's mouth; simply push the baby towards you.

6. You should now have a happily latched baby (hopefully)

7. Consider looking at online videos of babies latching; there are lots of beautifully made how-to guides where you can see what is happening at each step. Don't be afraid to call a breastfeeding helpline; they are skilled at improving latching over the phone with you.

It Will Come Naturally

It almost makes me laugh how, on the one hand, you are told "breastfeeding is painful," while on the other hand, someone says to you, "oh, it'll come to you. Don't worry; it's the most natural thing in the world, after all!" We can't win, can we?

You know what else is natural? Walking, talking, eating, and sex, yet we learned these skills. Breastfeeding is no different. Your baby has never breastfed before, and you have never fed this baby before. Even if you are an experienced parent who has fed many babies well beyond toddlerhood, you have still never fed this baby. You are both learning new skills, and just like any other skill, it often feels clumsy, confusing, or even overwhelming in the beginning. That's why those who work and volunteer in infant feeding support try to be as helpful as we can, and it's why we keep banging on about getting help for pain or weight problems. Sometimes, we need help to learn a skill and that is okay.

I took up knitting while the world was locked down in 2020. I was hopeless at it. I watched dozens of videos, bought various types of needles and wool, but I could not make it work. I just ended up in a frustrated, tangled mess every time. Then, someone took pity on me, and over Zoom, we spent an hour together. By the end of that hour, I had the tools to knit a wonky, holey scarf. I just needed the right support from the right person. Breastfeeding is often the same. Get the right support from the right person, at the right time, and you will be far more likely to meet your goals.

It Won't Matter If You Can't

Many parents tell me: "When I was pregnant, I said I would try to breastfeed, but I wouldn't get upset if it didn't work. So, why am I heartbroken at breastfeeding not working?"

I hear this most days. We forget that once the baby is born, our bodies make a huge hormonal shift needed to make breastfeeding work.

> *I just thought it would be something I'd try and if it didn't work, I'd give my baby formula instead. But after she was born, it was like a switch went in my head and suddenly, I had to breastfeed her. I still can't explain it today!* ◆ **Megan**

In addition to this, parents who've been through a difficult birth experience really want to make breastfeeding work. Often, mums will say to me, "I failed at the birth—I can't fail at this too."

> *I felt like such a failure for not birthing him naturally, the thought that I was also failing at breastfeeding was unbearable. Was I even meant to be a mother if I couldn't do these really natural things?* ◆ **Mel**

Then, we've got the sheer hard work that goes into breastfeeding. It can often feel completely unacceptable to give up after several weeks of battling challenges. I know several women who have simply dug their heels in with utter determination that they were going. To. Do. It. Because they had already given it so much, and couldn't stand the idea that they had worked so hard and not got what felt like a positive outcome.

Finally, parents often talk to me about the way their baby seems to enjoy breastfeeding more than bottle feeding, or that Mum herself finds breastfeeding especially lovely, or making bottles and buying formula is expensive or time-consuming. That's just a few of the reasons parents tell me they want to make breastfeeding work; the full list is so much longer.

Regardless of the exact reason, it is likely that, as chilled out as you are before your baby is born, this will change once that baby is in your arms. For this reason alone, preparing to breastfeed is a good idea.

You Will Have Problems If You Have a Cesarean

Someone somewhere seems to have taken a valid point about C-sections being a bit tricky for starting breastfeeding and turned it into this huge issue. Then, parents talk to me and tell me how amazed they are that everything was just fine after their cesarean. The myths here are threefold:

1. Your milk will be delayed coming in
2. It will be too painful to hold your baby to feed them
3. You/your baby will be too tired/traumatised to breastfeed

So, let's tackle these one at a time.

1. While studies tell us that caesareans lead to more issues in the first five days of breastfeeding (Evans et al., 2003; İsik et al., 2016), by day 5, these issues are resolving and breastfeeding can usually carry on. The challenges reported are milk becoming more abundant can be delayed by several days and that babies take less milk overall than their counterparts born by vaginal delivery. These issues don't need to be a big deal, though. Here are some tips for managing them:

    - If your caesarean is planned, hand express some milk before the baby is born and store it in your freezer. You can use this if your baby is sleepy, needs top ups, or your milk is delayed coming in.
    - Hand express after some feeds in the first few days, even if you think things are going well. You could feed this back to your baby on a teaspoon or in a syringe, or pop it in a fridge to be used later.
    - Keep your baby skin to skin with you and offer the breast often—every 2 hours in the day and 3 hours at night, but don't panic if they don't want to feed every time. It's common for babies born by caesareans to be a bit sleepy.

- Get help *early* if you are having problems. Remember that help may need to be outside of the maternity services you are under. Or you might need to see a specific person at the maternity unit/in the community health visiting team.

2. When I had my emergency caesarean with my youngest baby, Oliver, I remember thinking, "How am I going to keep those feet away from my wound?" The reality was that this was nowhere near the problem I had imagined it to be. There are many feeding positions we can try that keep little kicking feet away from that fresh wound low on your tummy. Cross-cradle, cradle, and rugby ball hold are the most common. Even if you wanted to try Biological Nurturing or side lying, this can usually be achieved comfortably with a folded-up towel acting as padding over your sore tummy. Breastfeeding pillows, or even just a regular bed pillow, can also act as padding while you're sitting upright to feed, if you are worried about feet finding their way down that low.

3. Once the medication wears off, a burst of hormones will hit that will make you feel super awake and entirely focused on your new baby. This is why so many people share photos of their first hours after birth. They're too elated to sleep. You might also feel tired and sore as well. This is why breastfeeding is great; you can do it in bed! It's also great for helping babies recover from birth because everything about your breast and chest feels like home to your new arrival. Even the fluid secreted by your areola has a smell that drives babies to feed (Doucet et al., 2009). Keeping your baby skin to skin for as long as possible in the first few days helps you and your baby feel safe, calm, and connected. It also helps breastfeeding to get established.

I was worried that my planned (necessary) section would mean that breastfeeding was harder, so I expressed my colostrum in the week before the big day. I ended up giving her 5ml on day 1 because she was sleepy, but apart from that, everything went well. My milk came in on the third day as normal, back to birthweight on day 10, and breastfed for 19 months. ◆ **Hollie**

If Your Mother Had Problems, You'll Have Problems

Here's another myth that could be true, but not for the reasons you might think. We often assume that lactation challenges are hereditary, but this just isn't backed up in science or lived experience. Your mum's experience of breastfeeding *can* impact yours, but because of her influence, not her handed down physiology. Let's share the stories of two mums as an example:

> Anna was breastfed for 3 years as a child. Her mum was a breastfeeding counsellor in the 90s and Anna was often exposed to new mums visiting her home for feeding help with their babies. She grew up surrounded by the normalisation of breastfeeding. She understood from a young age that babies feed a lot, and how a good feeding position looks. When Anna has her first baby at 27 years old, she already knows the basics of latching and feeding through a lifetime of osmosis. When she does have some pain or a worry, she asks her mum for help, and gets breastfeeding support for her breastfeeding problems.
>
> Zoe was not breastfed at all because her mum tried with Zoe's older brother for 3 weeks and found it too painful. If breastfeeding ever came up in Zoe's childhood, it typically involved her mum telling an anecdote about Zoe's brother "destroying" her nipples. Zoe helped to bottle-feed her younger sister when she was born, and like many of us, grew up in an environment where lactation was not discussed or normalised. When Zoe has her first baby, also at 27, she wanted to breastfeed. However, not only had she spent her childhood hearing how difficult it was, but throughout her pregnancy, her mum, keen to not let her daughter suffer like she did, bought her bottles, formula, a milk preparation machine, and books about routines for babies. Zoe finds breastfeeding painful, her mum validates that this is normal, and tells Zoe that formula was good enough for her so how about she doesn't worry about breastfeeding; it's not worth the pain.

Our parents want to help us, but often, they try to help from their own experiences and, with nearly all women in the UK during the 80s and 90s formula-feeding soon after their babies were born, it's not surprising that we grow up believing the women in our family just can't breastfeed. Not surprisingly, these women can't get help with breastfeeding when it's our turn 20+ years later.

You Will Struggle (or Get on Well) Because of the Colour of Your Skin or Hair

This is such utter nonsense that I struggle not to roll my eyes when someone tells me, "She'll have no problem breastfeeding because she's Black" or "My friend said it hurts so much because I have red hair." I would like to jump into the complexities of lactation for parents of colour, but that needs to be a book in itself, preferably written by someone with the history of such trauma flowing through their ancestry. I am able to say that our Black mamas may need more support and information than White mamas because they likely experienced systematic racism in their maternity care.

As for the red hair thing? I once supported a mum who dyed her hair a gorgeous natural-looking red. When her baby was born and she found breastfeeding painful, she was told this was due to the colour of her hair. Her excellent response was "Wow, I didn't know a bottle of hair colour had such an influence over my baby's latch."

There's No Point in Trying If You've Had Breast Surgery

Parents are often told that breastfeeding won't work if they've had breast surgery. Surgery *may* lead to problems but it certainly isn't guaranteed. In fact, many mothers breastfeed successfully with breast implants or even the usually more problematic breast-reduction surgery.

Breastfeeding with Implants

I usually ask mothers why they had implants. Women may have had breast implants because their breasts didn't develop as expected. This could point to underlying problem such as limited milk-making tissue. If their reason for implants is asymmetric or very small breasts, or breasts that looked unusual, then that might make it harder for them to fully breastfeed, but it certainly doesn't make it impossible.

- Next, I will ask where the incision for your implant was made. If, for example, the incision was made around your areola, it may be harder to breastfeed as nerves may well have been cut. You need full sensation to recognise that a baby is suckling. If your incision was underneath the breast (inframammary) or in your armpit (Axillary), then then your milk-making tissue, along with the important nerves, may have been preserved and you can produce a full milk supply. Other methods of surgery can also damage milk-making tissue, or important nerves, but these should be considered on a case-by-case basis. Adopting a "wait and see" approach may be your best option in regard to breastfeeding.

Breast-reduction surgery is more likely to negatively impact your milk-making potential than implants, but there are still a few things to consider regarding your chances of breastfeeding after breast reduction:

- The type of surgery is important. Liposuction is the least damaging type of breast reduction, as it only removes fat and leaves the ducts and nerves intact. The inferior pedicle technique (sometimes called the anchor technique, as it leaves an anchor-shaped scar around your areola) leaves a lot of tissue connected so causes less damage than the other methods, such as periareolar.

- Next is how long ago you had the surgery. Breast tissue can regenerate. The more time that has passed, the better. It takes about 5 years for nerves to repair.

- While you may find it hard to make a full milk supply if you've had a breast reduction, it is not impossible, and it is important to remember that *any* human milk benefits you and your baby; it's not just nutrition. Feeding at your breast comforts and feels safe for your baby, for as long as you and they want to continue.

Even if a full milk supply is not possible, breastfeeding should not be dismissed. It's often worth a wait-and-see approach. Remember, *any* human milk is beneficial to tiny humans.

If You See an IBCLC, They Will Force You to Breastfeed

An IBCLC (International Board-Certified Lactation Consultant) is globally considered to be the expert in infant feeding. Yes, breastfeeding, but also formula-feeding. We regularly support parents to use formula or donated milk when babies need some extra help, or the parents don't want to exclusively breastfeed. An IBCLC who makes you feel pressured or forced into breastfeeding only, especially when extra milk is medically indicated, is not meeting their ethical or professional requirements to ensure that a baby is fed appropriately. IBCLCs also need to support families in making decisions that are best for them, not the lactation consultant.

Anyone Can Call Themselves an IBCLC. It's No Big Deal

Anyone can call themselves a lactation consultant, but the title IBCLC (International Board-Certified Lactation Consultant) is protected. In addition to this, IBCLCs undergo significant levels of education and training before qualifying. The profession dates back to 1985, when the first exam was administered. Since then, the exam has been available once or twice per year all over the world, with over 26,000 candidates since 1985. IBCLC is the only internationally recognised qualification in lactation, and it is independently accredited. The International Board of Lactation Consultant Examiners (IBLCE) keeps a registry of all qualified IBCLCs. You can search for someone by name to check they are as qualified.

An IBCLC must uphold several responsibilities, which someone calling themselves a lactation consultant may not be bound by. These include:

- Be an advocate for breastfeeding as the norm
- Educate professionals, families, and the community about lactation
- Give comprehensive, evidence-based information and skilled support from before conception through to after the child weans
- Help to develop policies that protect and promote breastfeeding
- Perform and document thorough feeding assessments
- Communicate with other members of the healthcare team
- Focus on family-centred care and counselling skills to support families to reach their infant-feeding goals
- Provide appropriate follow-up care

Becoming an IBCLC is no easy task. It typically takes a minimum of 2 years, with requirements including:

- Either a medical background or the completion of 14 health science courses at college level
- 1,000 hours of experience supporting families with breastfeeding.
- 90 hours of additional lactation-only education
- A 4-hour exam
- Maintaining their qualification by submitting Continuing Education Recognition Credits every 5 years.

Don't Trust a Breastfeeding Advocate; They Are Only Interested in Your Baby Being Exclusively Breastfed

A few people, typically on social media, are vocal about what they call "desperate Formula-Feeders." The conversations in these spaces tend to be along the lines of "but why don't people try *harder*?" However, once someone has been involved in breastfeeding support for more than 5 minutes, they quickly lose that attitude. A lot of breastfeeding supporters have come into their role because they had a hard time breastfeeding. They often combi-fed, stopped breastfeeding before they wanted to, or ran into other problems along the way. They are usually trained in parent-centred support (which means what you want, and need are the only things that matter, safeguarding issues aside), and they are taught counselling and active listening skills. You might come across the occasional overzealous new recruit, but it is unlikely. Please, give a support group or drop-in a try before you stop breastfeeding. It could make all the difference, and you may even make friends for life.

You Can Only Get Support from a Breastfeeding Advocate/Supporter If You Want to Carry on Breastfeeding

People trained in breastfeeding support are trained in *all* areas of human-milk feeding, including how to support parents with stopping, whether that might be after a couple of feeds or several years. You should always get non-judgmental, kind, and understanding support from a breastfeeding volunteer or professional when you go to them for support with ending your breastfeeding relationship.

CHAPTER 3

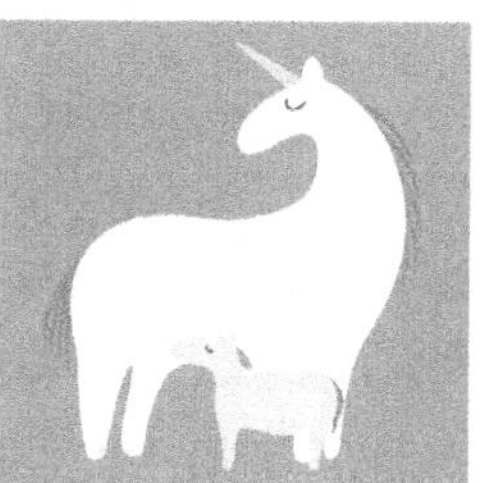

Breastfeeding Life with Your Newborn

Colostrum Is Not Enough

This idea has been around for a long time. In fact, in some cultures, colostrum is discarded, and babies are given glucose water or some other concoction in the first few days of life because colostrum is seen as dirty or unhealthy. Some cultures require mothers to bathe at home before they can begin breastfeeding their babies. Here in the West, we think that mothers go from 5ml of colostrum on day 1 to a full supply on day 3, and there's nothing in-between. If you don't see your colostrum, and your baby is latching to feed hourly, we become convinced that there is no milk in our breasts at all. Add to this the fact that many babies are being readmitted to hospital around day 3 to 5 with jaundice or dehydration, and we can easily jump to the conclusion that colostrum isn't enough milk for a newborn.

The flaw, however, is that colostrum isn't the problem: lack of breastfeeding information and support is. The *biggest* reason babies don't get enough milk in the first few days is that they aren't removing it often or well. Either they are latching poorly, or they are sleeping through feeds, and no one is helping the parents to identify these issues. I have become increasingly convinced that helping parents to hand express for a few minutes after three or four breastfeeds a day until milk comes in, and either offering this to baby on a spoon or in a syringe, or storing the milk in the fridge, is the quickest way to ensure that babies are not readmitted to hospital on day 5. Expressing milk also encourages mums that they do have milk in their breasts because they can see it.

In addition, colostrum is more than nutrition for newborns. Most full-term, healthy babies are robust and don't need as much milk as we might think in the first day or so (Santoro et al., 2010); they've got stores of fat to keep them going while they figure feeding out. Colostrum is rich in secretory IgA, lactoferrin, and leukocytes, as well as developmental factors, such as epidermal growth factor. These ingredients support the immune system, protect the gut, and help a new human transition to life outside of the womb.

So, is there any truth to this myth? In some cases, but it's usually a feeding issue, not a colostrum issue. Get support early, and if you're still worried, hand expressing after a few feeds to give the milk back to baby will often keep things ticking over nicely.

Your Baby Is Feeding Too Much

Tell me, over the last 24 hours, how many sips of water have you taken? How many cups of coffee? How many snacks and meals? Tastes of a recipe you're preparing? How many chips pilfered from someone's plate? Assuming my own routines are average, you're probably looking at several glasses of water, a few hot drinks, three meals, and a couple of snacks. Then a biscuit. Or three.

We often say that babies should feed eight times in 24 hours. What we forget to mention is that this is the *minimum* number of feeds expected. When we consider how often adults eat and drink, that suddenly becomes a whole lot more relatable. As adults, we'd struggle if we could only eat and drink in perfect 3-hour intervals. Yet our babies, who are tiny and vulnerable, with little stomachs, are expected to fall into a routine that ties in with our modern need to sleep all night and work outside of the home (without a small human strapped to our back) all day.

Babies feed a *lot*. Adults feed a lot, too. Toddlers are eating machines, as are teenagers. Your baby also wants to feed often. Very often. They are not broken, but let's consider some warning signs that feeding may not be going well. Breastfeeding hurts and your baby,

- Is not gaining weight in a way the professionals around you are happy with
- Has jaundice in the first 48 hours of life
- Is not pooing daily in the first 6 weeks of life
- Is not producing lots of heavy wet nappies every day
- Is consistently difficult to wake up
- Is either feeding or screaming/crying, and this seems to be happening all day, every day
- Sleeps through the night from a young age, and weight gain is a concern

Your Baby Must Have Formula Top Ups

If your baby has lost more than an ideal amount of weight or they are slow to gain weight, your provider will likely suggest top ups. Many people assume that these top ups need to be of formula milk. However, often, it's possible to pump and give your baby breastmilk. In the meantime, it's important to address *why* your baby is struggling to remove enough milk from your breast. While low supply is possible, if your baby is 2 weeks old, the problem is likely something to do with latching. A thorough breastfeeding assessment, breast compressions, and switch nursing can all significantly increase milk intake before we begin to top up.

We should also consider donor milk. Feeding your baby someone else's milk is something many of us in the West are uncomfortable with. However, human milk is so significant that the World Health Organisation tells us that if Mum's own milk isn't available, then donor milk should be considered before formula.

In the UK, it's difficult to access milk from a human milk bank unless your baby is premature or poorly. Lots of families informally share milk from friends, family, or via online groups.

In summary, if you're told to top your baby up, find out if this can be your own milk pumped, and if not, consider if you can access donor milk. Work on the issues leading to the slow weight gain (usually, these are due to your baby not feeding as well as they should be. These challenges can often be improved with good help and a bit of time.

Your Baby Is Okay to Lose 10% of Their Birthweight

This one always has me scratching my head. I think it probably falls into the mistake many people make about babies, which is trying to make them one-size-fits-all. For some babies, a 7% or even 10%weight loss on day 5 is totally okay. They're weeing, pooing, engaged with the world, swallowing beautifully at the breast, a lovely colour, and the mama is not in any pain. In contrast, when some babies lose 7% on day 5, alarm bells should be ringing. They are sleepy, jaundiced, Mum's nipples are all but hanging off, and there has been no poo for 36 hours.

It's common for doctors to tell parents not to worry about their baby's weight loss until it reaches 10%. As is often the case, the reassurances are designed to comfort. However, parents are often surprised when their babies are weighed on day 7 and they are told their baby *must* be readmitted *now*. It would be so much better if support was consistently given on day 5 and someone could tell if things looked a bit off. What might that support look like?

- A feeding assessment to check that your baby is latching well and swallowing consistently at the breast.
- Checking that Mum is not in pain.
- Checking that wet and dirty nappies are as expected (six or more heavy wet, and at least two dirty per day)
- Teaching the parent to hand express after feeds and to either feed this back to the baby or store it in the fridge in case things take a turn for the worse later. (We don't usually need to be getting out

a breast pump and forcing 15 minutes of expression after *every feed* at this point. But a few drops of extra milk through hand expressing a few times daily may keep things on track.)

If you're not sure how well your baby is doing on day 5, despite reassurances or suggestions to wait a couple more days before acting, then you may find it helpful to ask your healthcare professional to go over the above suggestions with you or you might want to seek support from a helpline/peer support group/IBCLC.

The Weight Charts Professionals Use to Track Weight Gain Are Based on Formula-Fed Infants

This is often used to demonstrate that we worry needlessly about baby weight gain. If your baby is slow to gain weight, someone will probably tell you the weight chart isn't accurate for your breastfed baby. This is no longer true. In much of the world, we use the World Health Organisation's standard charts to track weight gain in babies. These charts are based on a huge study called the Multicenter Growth Reference Study (MGRS) and they were released in 2006. The MGRS looked at over 8,000 children between 1997 and 2003 from all over the world, and these children were all breastfed either exclusively or nearly exclusively for a minimum of 4 months, and then breastfed alongside solids at least until they were 12 months old. The charts we use because of this study allow for babies to be slightly leaner and taller than we used to track previously. Most countries in the world now use the WHO standard charts, including the USA and the UK.

Don't Worry About Your Baby's Slow Weight Gain—Just Feed, Feed, Feed!

This myth frustrates me hugely and is usually seen in breastfeeding support groups online. If a baby is genuinely struggling to gain weight through exclusive breastfeeding, continuing ineffective feeding is only going to make it harder for them. I often see parents who come to me when their babies are 6 weeks old and only slightly above birthweight. The baby goes to the breast and quickly falls asleep. When I carry out an oral assessment, the baby's suck appears to be weak and disorganised. The parents report that things have gotten worse as the weeks passed.

We start a feeding plan including no more than 30 minutes of at-breast feeding and then a top up of either expressed milk, donor milk, or formula. I see the baby a week later and they are no longer falling asleep at the breast. the suck feels stronger, and the weight is up.

Why is this? When babies breastfeed, they use calories and energy. If they aren't getting calories back, they lose strength. Breastfeeding becomes harder for them because when they are weaker, they remove even less milk. The supply down regulates. There is less milk available for the baby who is already struggling. We end up in a vicious cycle of slow weight gain and a baby who is either crying or asleep. Even if we improve positioning and attachment at the breast, the baby will still struggle because the supply is likely reduced after weeks of milk not being removed consistently. So, we introduce a plan to gain strength, increase milk supply, and turn that vicious downward spiral into a positive upward one. If we just carried on with "feed, feed, feed," things usually do not improve because the baby is struggling.

If Your Baby Won't Latch, You Must Give Bottles

> *My little boy has never taken a bottle! The first few weeks, we did top ups (he lost 15% weight and my milk hadn't fully come in due to an induction and traumatic delivery). I was told in hospital to give top up by bottle. Baby Boy was having none of it! But would happily take top up from a cup pr via syringe. He has always drunk from a cup.* ◆ **Laura**

Did you know that in some countries, bottles aren't routinely used? Feeding devices have existed for as long as we have had babies. Cups, bowls, spoon-shaped vessels, even the mum's own finger have all been used to supplement babies who have problems with at-breast feeding. A mentor once told me about her grandfather who was fed with a teaspoon for the entire time that he needed breastmilk. His mum would hand express into a bowl and feed her baby the milk one slow spoonful after another, for months.

In the West, we tend to associate bottles with babies. While bottles are culturally normal and easy to access, they may not be the best way to feed your baby if you want to combi-feed. Bottles can make some problems worse. These are mostly to do with jaw and face development. In addition, babies fed with bottles are more likely to be overweight in later life, due to the way adults can override the baby's satiety signals by overfeeding them (von Kries et al., 1999).

Of course, you can give a bottle, and most people do. You can reduce the potential problems by using paced feeding and by following your baby's fullness cues closely.

Paced feeding slows down bottle-feeding so that a baby is less likely to overeat or struggle to switch between breast and bottle. There are lots of great videos online demonstrating how to do this, but essentially, we try to sit the baby upright, snuggled in close to their caregiver, and we avoid filling the teat completely with milk. Some parents worry that leaving a gap in the teat can cause wind or gassiness, but we think the symptoms of this are more likely to be caused by a baby feeding too quickly or taking too much milk, which paced feeding avoids.

You have other options, too. You could feed your baby with a little medicine cup or an eggcup if they're newborn. You could also try a teaspoon. Some parents use a little feeding tube taped to their knuckle and do something called finger feeding. If your baby is older than about 4 months, you could probably skip the bottle altogether and try a free flowing Sippy cup or beaker.

All the above suggestions can help with oral development and avoid bottle preference if your goal is to have your baby at the breast as well. Also remember that most babies who struggle to latch do eventually go on to breastfeed if they are given the time and the opportunity.

I was told, "some babies just don't like to breastfeed and yours is one of them." That was day 3 and now, 21 months later, we're still feeding. Thank God, I trusted myself and not that support worker. I'd like to add this was in a breastfeeding clinic. You would think they would have proper training in breastfeeding. ◆ **Alice**

If Your Milk Isn't in On Day 3 You Won't Be Able to Breastfeed

Milk supply typically becomes more abundant about 72 hours after the placenta is delivered. However, if you're a first-time parent, your baby is early, you had a lot of medication in labour, or you lost a lot of blood after your baby's birth, then your milk becoming abundant might be delayed. Milk "coming in" isn't like pushing a lever on a water fountain. We don't go from nothing to full flow! On day 1, your baby will take about 5 ml. each time they feed, and then the amount of milk you produce slowly increases each day until somewhere between day 3 and 5, your body goes, "Oh, you're feeding a baby? Well, here, have all the milk!" That is super helpful, but most babies do just fine for a couple of days if your body is a little bit slow on the uptake.

If your baby struggles with a milk supply that's a bit delayed, there's still no need to panic. You can hand express after your baby feeds and give them this extra milk. If you hand expressed in pregnancy, you could use this stored milk now. If you've been removing milk after feeds, bring this milk out now to use.

Let's assume the worst happens. Your baby needs more milk than you can give, and they need it now. You can give some formula and still breastfeed. Just express for any missed feedings and make sure you're getting good help with your baby's latch. Chances are that in another day or so, you will be dripping milk everywhere.

My milk didn't come in on day 3 so I was told I wouldn't be able to feed. It came in at day 9, and we are about to hit our 1,000-day nursing milestone. ◆ **Rebekah**

Babies Don't Poo Every Day

This topic upsets people on social media. Posting about how babies need to poo daily in the first 6 weeks really gets people angry on my Facebook page. Parents will jump in and say that their babies only had a bowel movement twice a week and were totally fine, and that it's scaremongering to tell people poos should be happening so often. However, let's look at the science behind this.

In the early weeks of lactation, breastmilk has more of a protein called whey in it. Whey is fast to digest; it whizzes through the stomach, and as a result, makes babies poo lots.

Sometime around 6 weeks, milk changes composition so that it's more casein dominant. Casein is harder to digest, so it takes more time. Therefore, babies may well poo less often after this point. Yes, sometimes going only once or twice a week.

Now, some babies just don't produce dirty nappies as often as we expect, and this might be totally okay for them. However, a lack of daily, copious poo is a red flag. It should make professionals sit up and wonder, "Is this baby moving milk from the breast properly?" or "Is this baby's tummy working as it should be?" We should be finding out how weight gain looks, how content the baby is, what the poo is like when they do go, and if breastfeeding is going well. We shouldn't be shrugging and saying, "Oh, breastmilk doesn't produce waste, so they don't poo often." This is not true for most babies.

If your baby is younger than about 6 weeks and they are not producing at least two dirty, yellow poops per 24 hours, then you should be asking for a feeding assessment and a tummy check for your little one. If these things come back as okay, then yes, you might just have a "unicorn" baby but we must check.

Cluster Feeding Is a Sign of Starvation (and It's Just Lots of Feeding)

I'm often surprised when parents don't know what cluster feeding is. Mums will tell me during my volunteer time that their baby feeds well all day, but their milk "disappears" at 5 pm. Cluster feeding is usually a normal baby behaviour, but what is it?

Parents are often told that cluster feeding is a time (usually in the early evening) when babies feed lots of times close together. While this is true, it paints a bit of a rosy picture. Cluster feeding is often accompanied by a grumpy, fussy baby determined to chew on their own fists while crying about how hungry they are. They refuse to latch for more than 10 seconds at a time. If you've been told cluster feeding is frequent feeds, and then your own infant acts like the world is ending, you'll worry that something is wrong. Many parents conclude that Mum's milk has dried up, her breasts are empty, or she isn't making enough milk for her little one at night.

Actually, this behaviour is common. The milk available to your baby while your breasts are soft during these mammoth fussy sessions is high in fat. So, while there isn't much of it, it's incredibly rich. Over several hours, we tend to see the baby taking these tiny amounts of high fat milk, then crashing out and sleeping for longer than usual. Many parents worry this is a baby collapsing into sleep due to hunger, but it doesn't seem to be the case.

You might wonder why babies cluster feed. We aren't quite sure, but the most common theories are that milk supply is lower in the evening, so babies need to feed more often to get their needs met. Or it could be that babies are overstimulated by the end of the day so need to comfort feed. Or that they are filling up on fatty milk to aid the fast growth that happens during sleep.

I suspect the answer may be all of the above. An overtired baby seeking comfort from a breast producing small amounts of high fat milk to help them grow. One thing I am confident about, though, is that if your baby is gaining well, breastfeeding is easy during the rest of the day, you aren't in pain, and you're seeing plenty of wet and dirty nappies, then cluster feeding is rarely anything other than normal.

"The Latch Is Fine"

I hear this daily. Mum's nipples are cracked and bleeding, but apparently, several people have told her that the baby's latch "looks fine/great/perfect." If I was the type to bang my head against my desk in frustration, I'd have had a massive forehead-shaped dent in my desk ages ago.

Imagine that you're trying on some new shoes, perhaps the most beautiful shoes you have ever seen. When you do your awkward shoe-shop walk to see how they feel, well, they pinch, rub, and just feel awful all over. You tell the sales assistant, who looks at the shoes on your feet and says, "Well, they fit you perfectly!" I'm guessing you would leave promptly without the shoes, and wouldn't return to that store.

"The latch looks great!" is kind of the same thing, but you can't just go out and get a new boob if the one you have already doesn't fit well with your baby. Luckily for your breasts, things can be done to improve the pain you get when things aren't working too well. Get help from someone skilled in breastfeeding support as soon as possible.

The trouble is that lots of things could be happening inside your baby's mouth that we can't tell just by looking at the latch. It's also common for a borderline okay-looking latch to be described as great, or for someone to only watch part of a feed, missing the point where that beautiful-looking latch slips and you end up feeling like your nipple is being mangled by a small, angry dinosaur. So, it might be that you need a tiny adjustment. It might be tongue-tie, a high palate, an unusual sucking pattern, stiffness from the birth, a sleepy baby, or previous nipple damage causing your pain. These things need a good feeding assessment to figure out, not a quick glance in the first 2 minutes of a feed. I would go so far as to suggest that if someone tells you the latch is fine, despite you being in pain, find someone else to help you.

Flutter Sucking Is Your Baby Taking the Fatty Milk

Flutter sucking is what a baby does towards the end of a feed. They make tiny, fluttery sucks and stop swallowing. Mums are often told the vibrations of a flutter suck will draw down the thick, fatty milk from deep in the breast. As is often the case, there is some misunderstanding here. The baby *might* stimulate a let-down (a burst of milk) because of the stimulation they are providing. Because they've been at the breast for a while, that let-down will likely contain milk that's higher in fat than the beginning of the feed. However, flutter feeding itself is not your baby getting the fatty milk. If your baby is gaining weight well and is happy, and breastfeeding is comfortable for you, then you don't need to be too worried about the intricacies of this. You can pop your baby off if you need to at this point (although, they won't be super happy about it), or you can let them flutter their way to another let-down or to sleep.

However, if weight gain is slow, you might need to do some breast compressions to help your baby get more milk. You might also need to switch sides and/or pump to remove any leftover milk yourself. This all depends on your own individual circumstances, of course. It's best to get lactation support so that you'll be given correct information. What we don't want is for your baby to hang out at the breast indefinitely if they are struggling to gain weight well and are not able to replace the calories from flutter feeding with a big mouthful of milk.

Tongue-Tie Isn't a Problem

Believe it or not, some professionals are adamant that tongue-tie is a myth. I agree that we need to ensure that breastfeeding basics are optimised before taking a pair of scissors (or a laser) to a baby's mouth. I have also supported enough cases where tongue-tie was clearly a significant problem. The idea that tongue-ties are a myth is bizarre to me, and that's not just my opinion. Numerous studies on tongue-tie indicate that it needs to be addressed if positioning and attachment are optimised, and there is a restrictive frenulum there alongside painful nipples, slow weight gain, or any feeding issues at all. Snip it.

However, I need to be clear. A lingual frenulum (stretchy piece of tissue) under the tongue is normal anatomy, with 99.5% of babies having one in one study (Haham, Marom. Mangel, & Dollberg, 2014). It's not simply the presence of a lingual frenulum we look for in tongue-tie.

What sort of problems might a tongue-tie cause? Some examples:

- Painful breastfeeding for Mum
- Slow weight gain
- Low milk supply
- Mastitis
- Fussy feeding
- Frequent feeding
- Clicking at the breast
- Baby slipping off the breast (often described as "nipple feeding")
- Green poo
- Colic
- Misdiagnosis of silent reflux

What do you need to do if you think your baby has a tongue-tie? First, make sure you have excellent breastfeeding support: someone who spends a good amount of time with you, watches your baby feed, helps you change position or latching technique, and doesn't just tell you "the latch looks fine" if you're gritting your teeth and counting to ten to get through the pain.

Once more common issues, such as latch adjustment, have been ruled out, a full tongue-tie assessment is a good idea. Here lies another problem. In the UK, when I ask parents if their baby has been assessed for tongue-tie, they will say, "Well, so-and-so said that she saw him stick his tongue out, so there can't be a tie there." This is *not* an oral assessment.

A full assessment of your baby's mouth includes examination of:

1. **The Palate.** A normal palate is smooth and slopes gently. Some babies have what we call a high palate or a bubble palate. This often presents as a dome (one parent called it a dent when they described it to me recently) in the roof of the mouth, typically the right size for an adult finger to fit into. This high palate often presents alongside tongue-tie, and we think this may be because tongue-tie develops early in utero, meaning that limited tongue mobility in the womb affects the way the palate is formed.

2. **Peristalsis.** This is the little front-to-back waves a baby makes with their tongue while sucking. A baby who can't make these movements might be struggling because their lower frenulum that holds the tongue in a position doesn't allow for free movement.

3. **Tongue Cupping.** This means the sides of the tongue try to curl up to meet a finger (or a nipple). If they don't do this, it may be because the frenulum is holding the tongue down.

4. **Tongue Extension.** We need to see that the tongue can get out past the lower gum and cover the lip. Otherwise, when your baby is feeding, you will feel that hard, bony gum on your breast tissue rather than a soft, pillowy tongue.

5. **Resistance to a Finger Being Pulled Out of Your Baby's Mouth.** We hope your baby has enough strength and suction to try to pull that finger back in!

6. **Lateralisation.** This is where we see if the baby can move their tongue from side to side. We use a finger rubbed along the lower gumline to see if the tongue can "chase" it. Sometimes, babies can lateralise one way but not the other, for example.

7. **Can We See or Feel a Frenulum, and If We Can, Does It Seem to Be Problematic?** This is tricky, as so many babies do have a frenulum. We're looking for something short, thick, or tight, which is hard to describe to parents. Often, if your baby has lots of the other symptoms, we'd send you off to a tongue-tie provider anyway, and they make the final judgement call on this matter.

8. **Feeding Assessment.** Can the baby stay at the breast? Do they click? Do positional changes make feeding better for the mum and/or baby? What do Mum's nipples look like after feeding?

As you can see, there is so much more to these assessments than simply noticing a tongue sticking out.

When your baby has had a proper assessment, you discuss the benefits and risks of cutting a tie with your practitioner. While the surgery is quick, simple, and usually straightforward, it *is* surgery, so there are risks to consider:

- **Risk of Bleeding.** The practitioner is going to use a pair of scissors to cut tissue. There will be blood. Usually, this is a small amount and short-lived. Mouths generally heal quickly, and breastfeeding right after the procedure calms your baby (and the mum), while also providing pressure to the wound. Occasionally, however, babies bleed more, and a very few need to be hospitalised (this is rare). Many practitioners won't snip a tie in a baby who hasn't received their vitamin K, since vitamin K aids blood clotting. For most babies, frenotomy is their first experience of bleeding. If there's a blood clotting disorder, you'll know about it post snip.

- **Risk of Breast Refusal.** Breast refusal seems to be more common in babies who haven't successfully breastfed. Imagine the first experience of something being in their mouth equals pain. I'd probably want to keep my mouth shut for a few days after that, too. This is one reason babies aren't routinely checked for tongue-tie at birth. We want them to feel safe and happy with things (boobs, mostly) in their mouths before we bring out something sharp.

- **Risk of the Frenotomy Not Helping.** Sometimes, a tongue-tie snip doesn't seem to help. In some cases, it makes things worse.

Babies need to re-learn how to use their tongues and feed better.

We were told that we couldn't possibly have a tongue-tie because my son could stick his tongue out. Having someone tongue-tie trained disproved it, as he had very little useable range of tongue movement upon an oral examination. ◆ **Lauren**

Tongue-Tie Is the Cause of All Your Problems

Some people will tell you that tongue-tie isn't a problem. Others suggest that a frenotomy carried out ASAP will solve all your challenges. I wish this were true; it would be so easy, wouldn't it? A quick snip, and the problem is solved. Your baby is feeding well, no pain for the parent. Sadly, it's just not true. As I touched on above, consider the risks when deciding about frenotomy, including the risk that it might not improve things for you and your little one. More than this, though, tongue-tie is often a scapegoat for issues that frenotomy cannot solve.

If you've read this far, you won't be surprised to learn that things misdiagnosed as tongue-tie are usually related to positioning and attachment. Quite often, the parent is dealing with nipple pain and the baby isn't gaining weight well. The person supporting them runs out of ideas to help, so tongue-tie is suggested. Not surprisingly, many parents grasp at this as a possible quick-fix for their pain. They are then disappointed and frustrated when the tongue-tie practitioner tells them that there is no tie.

Positioning and attachment are not the only things to consider. Some babies are born with tension or tightness in their muscles that can make feeding difficult. For example, the cranial nerves in the base of the skull impact oral function. If a baby has arrived quickly, had the aid of forceps or a suction cap at delivery, or if they were just in an awkward position in utero, those cranial nerves might be causing difficulties. Fortunately, cranial osteopathy is widely accessible and considered safe. Some of my IBCLC colleagues strongly recommend that their clients see an osteopath before having a tongue-tie snip.

Some babies also just struggle to get a big mouthful of breast in the early days. Some people call this a poor fit: a horrible term I avoid. If there is a tiny baby with a small mouth, and a mum with comparatively large nipples, they might not fit together at first. This can cause pain, difficulties transferring milk from breast to baby, and slow weight gain. Breastfeeding techniques, such as breast shaping, can help in these cases, along with a little bit of patience while the baby grows, and breasts become less swollen.

If babies have a frenotomy before breastfeeding is positive for them, they can develop breast aversion, where they refuse to nurse after a tongue-tie revision. Obviously, this is stressful for parents and their babies. It's another example of why tongue-tie shouldn't be the first thing we address.

The take-home message here is to not jump to tongue-tie right away (unless it's obvious), but instead, make sure that you have had good breastfeeding support, that the problems are not better explained by something else, and that something less invasive won't help instead.

Lip Tie Is a Common Issue

This is such a tricky topic for me to broach to an international audience. In the UK, we rarely consider lip tie to be a problem, but I am aware that in the States, babies are regularly snipped, and parents report improvements in feeding. Let's dig into this topic with some anatomy.

The upper labial frenulum is a membrane that is commonly found under the top lip, in the middle. It's good at adapting to the way lips move, and as teeth come in, the mouth grows too, and the labial frenulum tends not to get in the way (Townsend et al., 2013).

Lip tie became something dentists in the US were keen to cut relatively recently, and this started because some people were worried that leaving some labial frenulum in place could lead to a gap between the teeth and possibly dental problems. Somewhere along the line, this has led to the theory that lip tie can cause feeding problems. The basis of this seems to be that people assume the top lip needs to flange outward during feeding, and the labial frenulum stops this from happening. However, studies have clearly shown us that this is not the case. We expect the top lip to remain in a neutral position during breastfeeds, so a flanged-out lip isn't ideal or expected, and actually suggests a shallow latch. I suspect that the reason we imagine a baby feeding with flanged out top lip as being normal may come from generations of watching them feed with bottles, where we do tend to see that sort of position.

Sarah Oakley (2021), in *Why Tongue-Tie Matters*, explains that lip ties are often cut at the same time as tongue-ties, and therefore, it isn't possible to say with confidence that the labial frenulum being released is what improved things. She discusses a presentation at a tongue- and lip tie conference. The speaker was Holly Puckering, a speech and language pathologist. She found that when she stopped dividing lip tie at the same time as tongue-tie and, instead, focused on tongue function first, the clinic's lip tie division rate fell from 22% to 1.3% in a year, with no problems reported for the babies or parents (2021, pgs. 129-130).

Interestingly, while lip tie revision is common in the US, in the UK, there are only two providers who will release them, and both are dentists, not infant-feeding experts. The same applies in the US; most lip tie practitioners are dentists, not feeding specialists.

You Need to Drink Milk to Make Milk

I wish this weird and nonsensical idea would drop off the edge of the Earth. How anyone spouting this nonsense thinks vegans, or those with cows' milk allergies, produce milk is a mystery to me. Most of Asia doesn't drink milk and still manage to breastfeed. This myth is either about the idea that milk comes from cows, so drinking cow's milk helps us produce more milk, or that we need a high protein/high calcium diet to produce breastmilk. This latter theory is slightly less insane than the idea that drinking milk from a cow makes us lactate.

Human milk is made from our blood, not our diet. That's why it protects babies' immune systems; its packed with white blood cells, not with the burger you ate last night, or the kale you ate for breakfast to try to undo the pizza. When we look at maternal diet and lactation in studies, the results are clear; you don't need to megadose on anything to lactate. Not cows' milk, not calcium, and not protein. You just need to eat a normal, well-balanced diet. Yes, that can include pizza.

We have evolved to keep our babies alive. If we needed to eat a block of cheese every day to achieve that, we wouldn't be successful at growing beautiful, chubby babies with all those leg rolls. We would have all the leg rolls, now that I think about it.

> *I was told that I needed to drink cows' milk to produce breastmilk. I'm vegan! We nursed for 3.5 years (16 months of breastmilk, then dry nursing for other reasons).* ◆ Jessie

Make Sure You're Eating a High-Protein Diet

Let's look at the issue around protein. Human milk is relatively low in protein at 0.8g per decilitre because babies don't need a lot of protein to grow. They require around 11g per day. Compare this to their intake of fat, which is 38g per day, and you can see the difference. Protein is good for fast bone and muscle growth, which is less important to human babies than their brain development, and, you guessed it, the brain needs plenty of fat to grow.

So, if your baby doesn't require a lot of protein to grow well, you don't need to be worried about eating lots of it yourself. Certainly, a diet lower in protein isn't going to impact the composition of your milk, so if you're craving carbs for those midnight feeding sessions, you can go ahead without worrying that you're negatively affecting your baby's protein intake.

Lactation Cookies, Teas, or Shakes Will Boost Your Milk Supply

The only people benefitting from "lactation-boosting" teas, shakes, and cookies are those who sell them. There is nothing wrong with eating or drinking these things (usually), but they will not help your supply. If you have a genuinely low milk supply, what you need is help to work out why and then appropriate support to increase it. Yes, that might include supplements sometimes found in the teas, but the doses you would need are stronger and more consistent (you might need tinctures or capsules). Getting your herbs that way will probably be cheaper, not masked with sugar, and you would be offered breastfeeding support alongside.

The commercial foods and drinks you can buy typically contain ingredients like:

- Brewer's yeast
- Flaxseed
- Oats

However, these active ingredients are usually lower on the ingredients list, meaning that they are present in tiny amounts. In one 45g, cookie I looked at, the first active ingredient, oats, was sixth (behind sugar, butter, wheat, egg, and chocolate), and flaxseed and fenugreek were present in the smallest quantities in the product, coming in last on the list.

For comparison, doses of fenugreek recommended for increased milk supply are typically 3,500mg-7,000mg per day, taken as several 500mg capsules. In addition, as you can see in the section below this one, fenugreek isn't super effective as a milk boosting herb anyway. (Hint: Neither are oats, flaxseed, or brewer's yeast.)

Oats may help a little bit, though no one seems sure if this is a placebo to do with the association of comfort, leading to an oxytocin surge, or due to the high(ish) iron content in them. Flaxseed, too, might be a bit helpful, but there is little research out there that I can refer to here.

I'm not one to dismiss what parents say is helpful. I believe that when parents are relaxed and feel proactive, breastfeeding goes better. However, I do get cross when mothers are sold these expensive products without good evidence, and with limited levels of the so-called active ingredients. If you want to boost your supply, specific food and drinks won't do anything without good lactation support, and you'd be far better off spending your money on a lactation consultant (who can refer you to someone who can recommend effective herbs, medications, and supplements if actually indicated.)

Fenugreek Is Great for Milk Supply

Ah, fenugreek. The herb that is seen as a magic bullet for breastfeeding problems. Fenugreek has a long history as a galactogue in many parts of the world, but there is not a lot of evidence that supports its use. Yet, it remains immensely popular. If someone on social media asks for help with boosting their supply, fenugreek will be suggested in the first five comments. If there is genuine low milk supply, fenugreek is unlikely to help.

Fenugreek is a plant from the same family as peas, typically found in India. It's used as a culinary herb around the world and is used to make fake maple syrup. For lactation, fenugreek is sold in special teas, as well as capsules filled with powdered fenugreek seed.

Recent studies have found that for some people fenugreek, is "mildly lactogenic" (Lactmed, n.d.). Some studies claim it is effective, while others say it doesn't do much at all. Fenugreek also makes your sweat and urine smell like syrup. You can also have nausea and loose bowel movements. People who are allergic to legumes can be allergic to fenugreek. Fenugreek is also known to lower blood sugar levels, so it is not advised if you have diabetes.

The bottom line is that no herb or pill increases milk supply if your breasts are not being emptied well and often. If your baby is gaining weight well and mostly content at the breast, then you don't need medication (even if herbal) to increase your supply. If you have real issues with slow weight gain or troubles getting your baby off of top ups, fenugreek is not a magical fix. We need to work out why your supply is low and deal with that, not just stick an ineffective and unpleasant smelling plaster over the problem.

Your Milk Makes Your Baby Colicky

Your milk flow, or your breastfeeding technique, *might* contribute to your baby's colic. There might be something in your milk, such as bovine proteins from your love of cheese, but your milk itself probably isn't an issue. Human milk is designed to perfectly meet the needs of human babies. It doesn't make sense that it would lead to colic. Breastmilk is a clear fluid, as gentle on the tummy as water (one of the reasons we encourage you to keep feeding if your baby has a tummy bug). It's made up of hundreds of ingredients, many of them immune protective, alive, and important for all areas of growth and development. Interestingly, when breastmilk is thought to cause colic, the alternative suggested is formula milk: a cows' milk-based product with neither immunity support nor living factors. No compositional changes according to your baby's age, environment, or bacteria exposure.

So, lets discuss what might be happening instead.

Your Flow Is Too Fast or You Have an Oversupply.

If your baby is being hit with a fast flow of milk, this can be hard for them to control and can lead to tummy ache, as the milk reaches the stomach at a fast rate. This can manifest as crying, fussing, breast refusal despite hunger cues, green poop, and all over misery.

Your Baby Is Allergic to Something in Your Diet That Is Passing into Your Milk.

Dairy and soy products are the usual culprits here, but a few mums find that they need to eliminate other foods, such as eggs or wheat. A true allergy is unpleasant for all involved—screaming, bloody, mucousy, often green nappies, rashes, dry skin, snot—obvious pain for baby. The good news is that eliminating the allergen from your diet eliminates symptoms in your baby. Giving them formula often makes symptoms worse because the allergens in standard infant milks are more concentrated than in human milk.

A nurse told me that my son's "wind" wasn't due to CMPA/tongue-tie, as I suspected, but was due to me making "fizzy milk," as I was drinking too much soda water. Baby had tongue-tie until 17 weeks because nobody listened. He also had CMPA. ◆ **Heather**

Your Baby Has a Tongue-Tie

Tongue-tie can cause colic-type symptoms due to the way your baby struggles to take milk. We often see gassiness, distress, and even vomiting after feeds in babies with an oral restriction.

I had so many doctors tell me my baby had "colic" and that there was nothing I could do but wait 'til she grew out of it?

Colic isn't a diagnosis. Colic as people refer to it is a symptom of some other issue. For us, it was oral ties. Once they were revised, the fussiness, gassiness, and screaming for hours at a time magically disappeared! I trusted my gut that I knew my baby best, and just kept digging 'til I got to the bottom of it. ◆ **Claire**

Your Baby Is Behaving Normally

- We have such funny ideas in the West; babies should be put down, self-soothe to sleep, and not feed too often. Conversely, that crying is always a problem. Many babies in the fourth trimester are unsettled because they need parental physical contact and aren't getting it. Or they need to cluster-feed and are being asked to wait until it's been 2 hours. Or they are just exercising their right to express their feelings about, well, who knows, really? I guess I'd be pretty annoyed too, if I was trying to get used to big, wide, cold, bright world after 9 months in a dark, constant space. Sometimes, all we can do is put them in a sling or hold them in our arms and just ride it out with a good Netflix boxset and a takeaway.

You might wonder how to tell if your baby is acting normally or not. These checklists should help you:

Probably Normal

- Baby is content most of the day, but has a few hours where they are fussy
- Weight gain is on track
- Wet and dirty nappies are as expected in frequency
- Poos are yellow in colour, may be liquid in consistency
- Breastfeeding is not painful for parent
- Baby feeds calmly and copes well with the flow of milk

Needs Further Investigation

- Baby spends much of the day fussing or crying
- Baby is hard to feed
- There is blood or mucous in dirty nappies
- Painful feeding for mum
- Eczema, dry skin, or unexplained snuffles that don't go away
- Frequent green poo
- Baby gulps, splutters, or chokes on the flow of milk often

Seek Support from a Breastfeeding-Friendly Practitioner/Doctor

Working out the cause of these problems is like a puzzle. You likely need someone to watch a breastfeed in its entirety, and to take a full medical history from the breastfeeding parent. They should have a solid understanding of allergy symptoms in babies. Lots of parents will see different professionals for each part of this puzzle: an IBCLC for feeding support, a dietician for diet changes, and a doctor for the medical management or diagnosis.

You Need to Get Your Baby in a Routine as Soon as Possible

This suggestion always makes me wonder if the advice giver has ever had a baby. Newborns have no idea about time. All they know is if they feel hungry or full, comfortable or uncomfortable, safe or in danger. They have these amazing primal brains geared up for nothing more than survival. Parents responding to their cries helps their brains to develop over time (Lagercrantz, & Changeux, 2009). Our survival-brained babies aren't going to have the foggiest clue what a routine is or why you're trying to get them on one. They cannot rationalise or understand ideas like waiting for food or going to sleep when an adult decides it's time for bed. They are fuelled purely by their own internal systems. You could try to get your baby into a routine, of course, and you might find they seem to be okay with this for a while. However, at some point, babies change when they want food and sleep, and all this change makes parents think that they're doing something wrong. In reality, babies know what they need and when.

The risks of routines include missed feedings leading to reduced milk supply, distress for the baby and parents, including raising babies' stress hormones (BASIS Online, n.d.). Other risks include loss of parental confidence, and sleep problems later on in childhood (Bugental, Martorell, & Barraza, 2003).

We started to believe that babies need routine during the Victorian era and it grew in popularity as formula-feeding became more normalised.

Let's be honest, a predictable baby is easier to care for, especially if you have three other children and a job to deal with. We now understand that babies have no control over the timing of their needs and denying them these needs is significantly problematic, as well as stressful for the parents.

> *I was told that, in order to "effectively breastfeed," I needed to only feed every 4 hours and that I had to leave my baby to cry for 5/10/15 minutes before feeding to extend the time between feeds until we got on that 4-hourly schedule. We carried on feeding responsively and fed until just after his 3rd birthday.* ◆ **Lauren**

Dad Needs to Give a Bottle So He Can Bond with Your Baby/Feel Included/Help You

Babies are designed to bond with one main caregiver first, and then to bond with more people over time. Everything about Mum is designed to make a baby feel safe and relaxed. Her smell is familiar, her heartbeat and breathing sounds were heard in the womb, her areolas secrete a substance that smells like amniotic fluid, and her breasts meets all nutrition, hydration, pain relief, and comfort needs. No other mammal expects the father to feed their young to bond, and many non-Western cultures don't have this expectation.

Having said that, it is lovely that, in the 21st century, fathers want to be more involved, but the idea that the best, or only, way to do that is with a bottle of milk is extremely flawed. To give that bottle, one of two things needs to happen with an already exhausted mum:

1. She Needs to Express Her Milk

This involves sourcing, setting up, learning how to use, and then using a breast pump for anywhere between 10 and 30 minutes. She then needs to store her milk, and wash the pump parts. When Dad gives the baby the bottle later, Mum's breasts, which are in tune with the baby's needs, won't get emptied. This can mean that she needs to go through the pumping rigmarole again to avoid getting mastitis.

2. **Dad Needs to Give Formula**

This often results in Mum feeling guilty, anxious about preparation, the volume of milk, or the baby's reaction. On top of the above, unless the baby is pace fed, they will possibly down the bottle of milk and then still look hungry, planting a seed of doubt that Mum isn't producing enough. We also risk bottle preference if the bottle is given often.

So, we can see that having Dad or the partner give a bottle of milk isn't as simple as it sounds. Thankfully, there are some wonderful things that partners can do instead, and no, that doesn't just include changing nappies.

- Wear the baby in a sling
- Hold the baby skin-to-skin
- Give the baby a bath
- Baby massage
- Cuddle the baby while Mum rests
- Take the baby for a walk
- Read to the baby
- Sing to the baby

All of the above are far more effective ways to bond with a baby because of the physical touch and communication involved. They can all keep your baby calm and happy for a few minutes or up to a couple of hours, allowing Mum time to shower, nap, or have some time to herself.

Finally, if possible, having skin-to-skin with your baby after birth was found to increase paternal bonding behaviours in a 2017 study (Chen et al., 2017). Dads who took part in this study had much higher scores when assessed for exploring, touching, caring, and talking to their babies on day 3 postpartum.

(I was told) That my husband would never bond with our son because he couldn't feed him. My son is now 15 months and doesn't want to know me when his dad is around. ◆ **Tanesha**

The Baby Needs to Get Used to a Bottle

While bottles aren't a particularly modern invention, we have had many ways of getting milk into babies throughout history, and many are still options today, including a cup, teaspoon, or a *paladai* (common in India). Once the baby is older than 4 months, you could introduce them to a beaker or Sippy cup. While bottles are socially acceptable and normalised in our culture, making them the preferred choice for most people, they do have downsides, including:

- Environmental impact (teats need replacing often, for example)
- Relatively complicated to clean compared to a cup or spoon
- Can cause problems returning to the breast
- It's easy to overfeed a baby with a bottle
- Oral development can be negatively impacted
- Higher likelihood of caries when used once teeth come through
- Some are expensive

Of course, if you plan to leave your baby for periods of time before they are 4 months old, particularly if you return to work and leave your baby in daycare, you will probably end up using bottles simply to avoid confusing caregivers and because you can also transport milk in a bottle. In this case, you don't usually need to give your baby lots of bottles in the lead up to this: two or three small bottle feeds a week, just so your baby knows what to do with it, is often all that's needed. However, if your baby refuses to take a bottle at all, that's okay! As discussed, it's not your only option.

Keep Feeds to 15 Minutes Per Side

I once heard a story from someone with grown children who now have their own kids. When she had her first baby, she had to feed for 1 minute per breast every 4 hours on day 1, 2 minutes on day 2, 5 minutes on day 3, and after that, she was to limit feedings to no more than 15 minutes. Apparently, the theory was that this would protect against sore nipples and stop the baby from comfort feeding. Her milk dried up.

Limiting or restricting feedings is a bad idea, but I still hear that feeds should last 15 minutes, or that you must offer the other breast after 15 minutes, or some other arbitrary version of this. Is there any evidence to support this? There may be some specific situations, but for nearly everyone else, there is no need to restrict feeding frequency or times. Think about it logically; every set of breasts is unique. Heck, even your boobs may differ: one makes loads of milk, the other makes less. We do not know how much milk a baby can take in 15 minutes if every breast makes a different amount of milk. Breastfeeding is not just about calories in, but also about comfort, pain relief, sleep support, temperature regulation, and bonding.

Limiting feeding time also prevents your baby from taking a full feed. The milk available starts out watery (but still important and nutritious), and as the feed progresses, your baby gradually takes more and more fatty milk. For some babies, they could reach that milk quickly and then happily come off the breast. For other babies, they might want to take their time and it could take them 30 minutes to get to the highest-fat milk. This is okay, but if we decide we know better and take the baby off after X amount of time, we could end up with a grumpy baby who wants to feed more frequently, which could lead to problems with milk supply. A study by Kent et al. (2006) looked at how often babies fed for and how feeding patterns determined fat and milk volume. They concluded that babies should be fed responsively, as often, and for as long as they want.

The only exception is if your baby struggles with weight gain and you need to give them top ups. You might need to limit time at the breast to 30 minutes before offering that top up. This is to prevent your baby from getting too tired to feed. The key is that you offer the breast again after the top up, and you use it under the guidance of qualified breastfeeding support.

Make Sure Your Baby Gets Hindmilk

Hindmilk is a word that's often thrown around support groups. "It could be too much foremilk. Make sure he stays on the breast for hindmilk at the end of the feed." There is a grain of truth in this statement, but it isn't something most parents ever need to even think about. Let me explain as best I can without a whiteboard and a set of markers.

Imagine a hot water tap. You turn it on, and, for a while, the water runs cold. Then, you feel it slowly warm up until it reaches its hottest point. Then, you turn the tap off. When you come back a few minutes later to use the tap again, the water won't be cold because some of the hot water will still be in the tap and it will reach the hottest point faster this time.

Your breasts are similar. When your baby feeds they taking what some people call foremilk, which has lots of water and plenty of other ingredients important for your baby's growth. As the feed continues, your milk slowly increases in fat content in the same way the hot water tap gradually warms up. If we take the baby off the breast before they are finished, they may not take the highest amount of fat available to them for that feed. If we put them back on that breast, they will take milk that is higher in fat, because the higher fat milk is still there. Basically, the softer the breast, the higher in fat the milk is. However, if babies feed as they need to—offering each breast, and then the first breast a second time—then most of the time, you do not need to worry about hindmilk.

Is your baby growing as expected? Are their dirty nappies yellow? Are feeds fairly faff free? If the answer is "yes" to all three, then keep doing what you're doing. The same is true, even if you are seeing occasional green nappies or a little bit of fussing for a few feeds each day. Remember, if something is a problem, it will happen most days.

If you are having problems with hindmilk, then it is likely not because of something you are doing wrong (unless you've been told to limit feeds to

10 minutes or something similar). Lactose overload (what happens when your baby consistently doesn't get enough fatty milk) is often a result of:

- A baby struggling to feed well
- Oversupply
- Timed or restricted time at the breast

You would know your baby was struggling with lactose overload because you would see:

- Green, explosive bowel movements
- A baby fussy at the breast
- A breast that still feels full after feeding

In this case, it would be a good idea to work with an IBCLC to figure out the underlying problem and treat it.

Foremilk Is Basically Water

Human milk generally has a high water content; it is a liquid, after all. Milk at the start of a feed is not just water, though. It is hydrating, but it's also full of lactose, vitamins, stem cells, antibodies, and fat too. Your body knows how to make milk that is right for your baby at that moment in time. It's clever. It would be wonderful if we could all trust our breasts to know what they're doing.

Your Milk Is Too Watery for Your Baby to Grow

Human milk has a thinner consistency than cows' milk or formula. However, it has everything babies need to grow, as long as you feed your baby every time they ask for a feed.

"You are making skim milk."

> *I was told this was the reason my daughter was having 8-10 loose stools a day at over 1 year old. I was told to stop nursing her because my "skim milk" was causing it. I knew better. Switched paediatricians. Turns out, she has an egg allergy and is lactose intolerant. I pushed for answers and referrals for GI for at least half a year and just kept getting blamed that it was my milk. My daughter was well in the upper percentage on weight too. She was healthy as could be, except her bowel movements.* ◆ **Brandi**

Your Baby Is Too Big; He Will Need Extra Milk

One reason why human milk is so awesome is that it adapts according to the baby's needs, including their size. The more your baby needs, the more milk they demand. The more they demand, the more milk you make. Your body is designed to feed twins, or even triplets. Many a 10lb baby has been exclusively breastfed with no trouble at all regarding milk supply. I want to turn this section over to the experience of parents, so what follows are several quotes that have come from the awesome mothers on my social media pages:

> *My second baby was born at 9lbs, 1oz and has been exclusively breastfed since birth. He'd lost 10% of his birthweight at day 3, but midwives were happy to let us carry on without top ups for a few days. By the time he was 10 days old, he'd regained his birthweight, plus a bit extra! The midwife commented that I'd done well, especially "feeding a bigger boy." I just followed my baby's cues and trusted in my body.* ◆ **Sam**

> *Third baby was over 9lbs. She fed immediately at birth and shortly after, and then went into NICU, where she was nil by mouth/not able to breastfeed directly for a while (lost over 10% of weight, unsurprisingly). When she was able to go directly to the breast again, she did so and then exclusively breastfed until 6 months, and carried on breastfeeding until about 3.5 years. No supply issues at all; I expressed while*

she was in NICE and started expressing again when she was about 6 months old to donate to a baby in need. ◆ **Meg**

I birthed five children, three of whom were 9.5 lbs. I exclusively breastfed all five children for about a year, and in the early months, they gained a pound a week. There was never any concern over my milk making or their milk transfer. I never doubted my abilities because I had the support of my family (all had breastfed) and LLL. They all self-weaned between 2 to 3 years. ◆ **Angela**

My second baby was born at 10lb, 2oz via crash C-section at 40+12. I was able to breastfeed him successfully until he was nearly 3, despite being told to give him formula when he was 18 hours old, because he was crying and disturbing others on the ward. He lost 3oz at day 5 and gained weight steadily after that. ◆ **Jemma**

If Your Baby Can't Latch in the First Few Weeks, Then They Will Never Breastfeed

This one makes me smile because my own baby latched for the first time at 18 weeks. If we keep the milk flowing and the breast available and safe, then usually, babies can figure out how to breastfeed. I have personally seen two babies latch for the first time at 1 year old. In both cases, the mum had pumped for them and then one day, the babies just spontaneously latched and fed. I have seen many more babies latch at 4, 5, or 6 months.

There are many reasons why a baby may need more time to latch, and these include:

- Trauma from birth
- Medication given to mum in labour
- Prematurity
- Cleft palate

- Down syndrome
- A high palate
- Tongue-tie
- Muscle or nerve tension

Most babies will go on to latch and feed, given time and opportunity.

If you have a non-latching baby, please don't panic. Here are some things to help them figure out what to do:

- Maintain a milk supply so that when the time comes, they have a reason to latch.
- Spend as much time as is realistic topless. If the milk makers are accessible and in sight, then there are a lot more opportunities for your baby to explore and latch.
- Keep your chest a safe zone. This means no forcing your baby to the breast, no pushing them while crying or arching their backs, and no shoving nipples into open, crying mouths in desperation. Instead, focus on allowing your baby to relax and rest a little higher on your chest, and when they are calm, by your breast itself. If we keep this area safe, then your baby is more likely to latch and feed eventually.
- Consider osteopathy or chiropractic to rule out tension or pain.
- Consider having a full oral assessment carried out by someone qualified to assess tongue and suck function (such as an IBCLC or tongue-tie provider).
- Some babies will latch with a nipple shield.
- Paced bottle feeding and skin-to-skin can be helpful in avoiding bottle preference.

Pumping Is Not Sustainable

Parents who have pumped long term will often tell you they found it easier than breastfeeding once they got into the swing of things. Pumping is predictable, for a start. You do it every two or three hours for 15-20 minutes (generally). Your pump doesn't cluster feed or get sick; it doesn't wake up every hour at night in a growth spurt. Your body responds consistently to that pump once it is primed to do so.

I'm not saying pumping is easy; it's just that those of us who have done it for an extended period know that it becomes normal to them. Normal usually equals sustainable.

There are challenges to exclusive pumping, including a need for consistency and effort when it comes to your pumping technique, as well as hurdles like pumps wearing out, electricity outages, pumping in public, and people asking you a lot of questions. However, for many parents, pumping is perfectly sustainable.

> *I got told only pumping would mean my supply would dry up by our health visitor. In the early weeks, they said if you don't get baby back to breast, it will dry up, as if it was down to me to get her to feed. No actual feeding support, though. Baby just couldn't latch but I knew my supply was there; baby just couldn't access it.*
>
> *So, it made logical sense to pump.*
>
> *I had read up online on how lactation worked so knew effective milk removal would mean that wouldn't be the case. I also bought the Stephanie Casemore book on exclusive pumping. It became my Bible! I stopped pumping at 21 months and sent an email when we reached a year to the health visitor team to tell them I had carried on pumping successfully. They never replied. This was in 2008.* ◆ **Zoe**

Pumping Reduces Your Milk Supply and Leaves Less in the Breast for Your Baby

Let's start this section with a quote from Nicky, who was told:

> *Pumping to provide top ups (because of poor weight gain caused by a tongue-tie) clearly isn't helping your supply because you don't seem to be producing much. Take 24 hours off pumping and make lactation cookies instead; there's evidence from studies to show that they really are effective at increasing your supply.*

You can hop over to the section on lactation cookies and supplements for more on that particular gem, but let's just remember how lactation works for a moment. The more you remove, the stronger the message becomes to make extra milk. Milk production depends on milk removals. If the baby is struggling to do this themselves (due to something like a tongue-tie as in Nicky's case), then a breast pump becomes the next best way to remove that milk. In addition, even if we leave aside the nonsense about lactation cookies for a moment and assume that they work, this would only be the case if milk was being removed. Your body will not keep making milk if milk isn't being taken out.

> *I was told when my daughter was 3/4 weeks old that exclusively expressing wasn't sustainable, as my body wouldn't produce milk without baby's latch. I was told this by a GP. We went onto exclusively express for 15 months.* ◆ Colette

Pumping Doesn't Require Any Special Technique

Around 98% of mothers express their milk at one time or another (Clemons & Amir, 2010). I reckon if you asked them, most would say that pumping was difficult. Typically, parents report that they are unable to remove enough milk with a pump, although this isn't always an accurate picture. Things such as the last time your baby fed, how good the pump is, and whether your baby is overfed pumped milk from a bottle all contribute to what "enough" actually means. However, pumping is typically harder than breastfeeding to manage.

There are several tips and techniques we can implement to help a mum remove more milk, and these seem to work in most cases, meaning that there absolutely is more to pumping than just sticking the shields on and turning up the power.

Warm Compresses Before Pumping

Yigit et al. (2012) found that more milk was removed when parents used a hot compress on the breasts before expressing.

Use the Pump's "Let-Down" Function Until Milk Flows

Some evidence suggests that pumps with a let-down function get milk flowing in around 90 seconds. Older studies found it took 4 minutes to get milk flowing with a pump. However, this research was carried out on one brand of pump.

Hands-On Pumping and Breast Massage

Morton (2017) tells us that massaging the breast while pumping yields significantly more milk than pumping alone.

Warmed Pump Shells

Kent et al. (2011) found that mothers removed more milk at the 5-minute point when pump shells were warmed before use.

Food/Drinks Mothers Were Told to Avoid While Breastfeeding

Before getting to the list, I should acknowledge that there are differences in cultural beliefs that we need to respect. This list is light-hearted and from a Western perspective, but if your culture dictates that you need to avoid certain foods, then that is entirely understandable.

For example, in some parts of the world mothers need to avoid hot or cold foods. It would be culturally inappropriate for mothers to ignore this. In the same way, different cultures have foods mothers are encouraged to eat in the postpartum period to support recovery and milk supply.

These are some foods that mothers reported that they were told to avoid. In most cases, it is not necessary.

> *I was told by a pharmacist that my daughter was constipated because I was drinking squash. I felt awful, gave it up (for the first time in my life), and my daughter went on to deal with chronic constipation for the next year.* ◆ **Charlie**

> *Spicy food, because baby won't like the taste of my milk.* ◆ **Ebony**

> *Fizzy drinks—they'll make your milk fizzy and baby gassy.* ◆ **Ebony**

> *I was told not to eat cucumber because it would make my baby colicky.* ◆ **Caroline**

> *Peanuts would apparently give my baby a nut allergy.* ◆ **Sophie**

> *I was told that strawberry seeds could pass into my milk and baby could choke on them.* ◆ **Laura**

> *Bitter apples. Specifically bitter ones. No idea why.* ◆ **Jo**

> *Onions would give her colic.* ◆ **Sarah**

> *Irn-bru sugar free will taint the colour due to being orange! But oranges are fine.* ◆ **Nicole**

> *Lemon cake; too acidic.* ◆ **Holly**

> *Orange juice with bits! Because the bits will come out with the milk, and they will give the baby diarrhoea.* ◆ **Megan**

> *Tomatoes would cause severe diaper rash due to raising the acidity levels in my milk and anything spicy would cause boob aversion.* ◆ **Macey**

> *I was told to avoid mushrooms because it's a fungus and will give baby respiratory problems. It was some randomer over social media though, so I definitely took that with a pinch of salt.* ◆ **Jessie**

A childless friend anecdotally told me of a woman he knew who drank blue WKD and consequently had blue breast milk. ◆ **Megan**

Broccoli; completely avoid it, said the GP, because it will cause trapped wind. ◆ **Joanna**

I was told to limit my liquid intake, drink just a little bit of water (if any), avoid soups and fruit in my diet, as I had an overproduction in the first months of my son's life. That should apparently help me to make less milk. I ignored this advice, as I did not want to die. ◆ **Renate**

CHAPTER 4

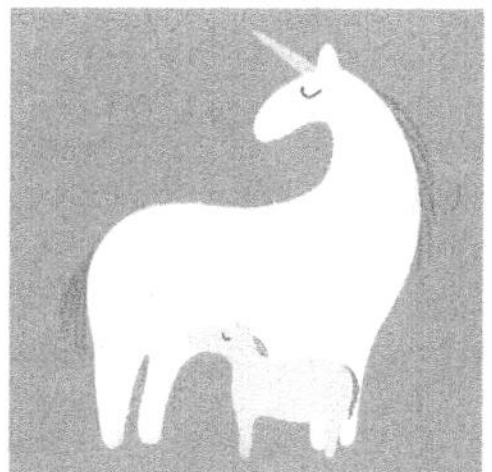

Breastfeeding in Months 4 to 6

You made it through the fourth trimester. Hooray! You may well still be ironing out some teething problems with latching, weight gain, or milk supply. If you fall into this category, please know that you are doing so well to still be giving your baby breastmilk, and that now, as you're halfway to starting solids already, things should start to get easier soon.

In this chapter, we'll be looking at many of the things you might hear people say between now and 6 months. One common myth might be, "Maybe your baby needs some solids early. You were eating chocolate pudding at 4 months and you're absolutely fine" (or a variant on that theme). Enjoy the evidence-based information here, and maybe eat the chocolate pudding yourself.

Your Baby Should Be Sleeping Through the Night

> *MIL: You should give baby some baby rice from 6 weeks to help him sleep.*
>
> *Me, EBFing: Baby slept 6 hours at a time by 6 weeks, and 8 hours at a time by eight weeks.*
>
> *(Then had normal sleep changes, but the food would've done nothing!)*
>
> ◆ **Rebecca**

Did you know that adults don't sleep all night? We tend to wake up, at least a little bit, to roll over, take a sip of water, use the loo, or elbow a snoring partner. We also only spend 6 to 8 hours sleeping. For some reason, we expect babies to sleep for 12 hours solid. This is one of those double standards that makes me pull an unflattering, confused face. Like adults, babies wake for many reasons. They're hot, cold, hungry, thirsty, scared, disorientated, have a wet nappy, an itch they can't scratch, they heard a noise, they're lonely, or they want a cuddle.

These reasons are all valid. You would wake up for the same reason. The difference is that you know how to go back to sleep. Babies haven't learned yet, and that makes so much sense. Having an adult close by at night keeps babies safe. From a SIDS perspective, but also from an evolutionary one. Imagine if your 6-week-old happily went to sleep anywhere in Stone Age times. You could pop them down, wander off to catch a mammoth or whatever, and you come back an hour later to find a sabre-toothed tiger licking his lips and no baby to be seen.

Your baby does not know that she is safe in her cot, being watched via a camera by her parents. Waking is normal and a great survival tactic.

Where does the myth of sleeping through the night come from? Primarily, Western culture. As far back as the Victorian era, male doctors were interfering in the work of childrearing, including infant care. The idea was that babies could be damaged if someone responded when they were crying. The quicker a baby could sleep for long periods, the better, as far as the West was concerned, and for various reasons, these ideas are still strong today.

You Can Force a Baby to Take a Bottle by Starving Them at the Breast

It's alarming how often I come across this, although it's mostly on social media rather than in the real world. This idea that a baby will take a bottle if they're hungry enough is, at best, misguided. Anyone who has tried to force babies to do something will know that hunger makes it *harder* for them, not easier. This myth also gets applied to babies who are struggling to breastfeed. Starving a baby into latching does not work. Babies feed best when they are calm and regulated. We need to offer milk often so they are not screaming with hunger that can lead to a 20-minute battle of trying to get babies to feed.

Supporting babies to take a bottle takes time and patience. Your baby needs to feel safe and comfortable with the bottle. Consider that a bottle is hard and cold, and that a breast is soft and warm. Also remember that babies are biologically driven to latch to a breast, not a bottle. The way their tongues move draws out milk from a breast and allows your baby to control the flow to some extent, at a speed they can cope with. A bottle is entirely different. The milk flows regardless of tongue function, regardless of hunger or satiety, and provides a lot less comfort than the closeness of Mum's heartbeat and scent at the breast.

Early Solids Will Reduce Frequent Breastfeeding

Human milk is high in fat and calories. Typical weaning food (carrots, for example) are low in fat and calories. If babies breastfeed frequently because they are hungry, giving them solids won't help that. In fact, some babies lose weight after early solids were introduced because, while their stomachs felt full, they weren't getting the nutrients needed to maintain their growth.

If babies breastfeed frequently for comfort or emotional needs, then surely, the last thing we want to do is give them food? In a culture where eating disorders, disordered eating, obesity, and body obsession are the norm, we should avoid programming babies to use food for comfort and emotional needs. The breast meets the need for closeness and connection, and hunger or thirst, without simply filling a stomach.

Soft Breasts Mean Your Milk Has Gone

Your body uses a lot of energy to produce milk. After it figures out how much is needed, it adapts so that less energy is wasted producing milk that isn't needed. In the early days, it's not milk making your breasts full. It's also inflammation and oedema. Once this settles down, most parents notice that their breasts start feeling soft again. By the time you're feeding a toddler, you might even feel that your breasts are empty, but your toddler will assure you otherwise.

The thing is, soft breasts work hard to make milk faster than full breasts. There's an ingredient in human milk called Feedback Inhibitor of Lactation (we often call it FIL for short). FIL increases as more milk is present in the breast. Its job is to regulate milk supply. Lots of FIL (full breasts) means that milk production slows, perhaps meaning that less milk is available later. When the breasts feel soft, less milk is available, so less FIL. This means that your breasts work harder and faster to ensure that milk is available for your baby.

Breastfeeding Makes Your Baby Clingy

Evidence suggests quite the opposite. Breastfeeding is the ultimate exercise in secure attachment. It means that every single need your baby has is met swiftly and consistently by a main caregiver. We know from the many studies that responsive and consistent parenting give children confidence to go off and explore the world, knowing innately that Mama will be there as soon as Mama is needed.

It might appear that this unique relationship is a clingy one, but it's exactly what nature intended and is perfect for growing brains. You may have seen breastfeeding babies or toddlers venture across the room before coming back for a quick check in and feed before they go off again. They don't need to cry to get their needs met. They don't have to look around and work out which adult is going to be most available. They just need Mum's breasts: consistently there, and the same, making exploration, and eventually, independence, safe.

You Need a Freezer Stash (The Bigger, The Better)

The increased desire for a freezer stash seems to come from social media, where mothers post photos of freezers packed with milk. That milk inspires something primal deep inside many mothers. It seems like a sound plan. What if you need to be separated from your baby? What if you have to go back to work soon?

It is unlikely that you will be separated from your baby for so much time that you need to leave behind a freezer full of milk. Even if you are going away for a weekend, you only need enough milk to cover the time you will be away, perhaps with a little bit extra to cover any spills.

The average breastfed baby takes about 750ml to 900ml of milk per day. This amount doesn't change from the age of 1 month until you introduce solids at about 6 months, when it starts to slowly decrease as your baby eats more food.

If you are separated from your baby, it won't be for more than several hours, perhaps for work, a medical appointment, or a spa day with friends. Babies can also adapt their feeding to take more milk when Mum returns. We call this reverse cycling and it's a great evolutionary way to ensure that the baby gets all their nutritional needs met, even if Mum has to be gone for most of the day.

There are some potential problems with having a large stash of milk. Some babies won't take milk that has been in the freezer. Excessive pumping can lead to mastitis, oversupply, a fussy baby, breast abscess, or nipple damage from a poorly fitted pump. A power outage can destroy a freezer stash in 24 hours.

I'm not saying you should have no milk in your freezer. Having an emergency stash can reassure you. However, your baby needs that milk more than your freezer does. Hours attached to a pump is not fun either, not when you could be snuggling with your baby. Pump if you're going away regularly. Don't stress if your stash is 500ml rather than 5,000ml. You're feeding your baby, so you're doing great.

Low Supply Is a Common Problem

I covered this in Chapter 2, but it's surprising how common low supply comes up again during the second 3 months of breastfeeding. Parents often feel that their babies are feeding more often, frustrated at the breast, and waking frequently because their milk supply is low. Pretty much anything a normal 4- or 5-month-old does might be blamed on milk supply.

People who suggest that mums have sudden onset low milk supply forget that a 4- or 5-month-old baby is different than a newborn. The world around them fascinates older infants who are easily distracted by a shadow, a light, or the cat. They can also become impatient at the breast, particularly if they sometimes have a bottle, or they prefer a faster flow of milk (like they get first thing in the morning). Frequent pulling off the breast, whingeing, fidgeting, or even hitting the breast usually means an impatient, distracted baby, not low milk supply.

Breast compressions help to maintain focus at the breast by increasing flow. You might also try offering feeds more often. You may need to feed in a quiet, low-lit, boring room. Some babies reverse cycle at this age too, where they feed more at night to make up for reduced daytime feeding. No wonder parents worry about supply!

Occasionally, you can experience late-onset low milk supply so if your baby is not gaining weight, you should be taken seriously. Hormonal contraceptives can cause of sudden-onset low supply, along with pregnancy. Some practitioners believe that as mother's supply settles down, a tongue-tied or otherwise struggling baby can no longer rely on a fast and copious let-down, and this may lead to slowed weight gain or similar issues.

It's Reflux

When babies are unsettled, the diagnosis is often reflux. Reflux is commonly diagnosed, with about half of babies having it. Reflux (aka gastroesophageal reflux disease or GERD) is a result of the stomach contents flowing back into the baby's throat. Endoscopy is when a scope is placed down the throat. It allows doctors to see if there is erosion of the oesophagus and is the only way to definitively diagnose it. Most GPs are understandably reluctant to do this and diagnose based on symptoms. For this reason, it is likely overdiagnosed.

Stomach acid, when it backs up into the throat, can burn or sting, causing unsettled behaviour, weight gain issues, or breathing problems. While these symptoms are on the extreme end on the spectrum for reflux, other symptoms, such as posseting milk after feeds, are common in infancy. The sphincter at the top of the stomach that stops its contents coming back up isn't tight enough to do its job well until around the time a baby can sit up.

Some possible symptoms of reflux include:

- Fussing at the breast
- A cough that doesn't go away
- A fussy/unsettled baby
- Slow weight gain
- Breast or bottle refusal
- Several incidents of vomiting daily (especially projectile vomiting)
- Pneumonia
- Lots of ear infections

Babies that are born early seem more likely to have reflux, and it might run in families.

However, these symptoms might also indicate a breastfeeding problem that requires skilled breastfeeding assistance, or that your baby is allergic to something like cows' milk. Fussy feeding, a distressed baby, slow weight gain, and feeding refusal can all point to latching difficulties, so get some skilled breastfeeding support before you resort to reflux medication. If your baby is using bottles, reduce the amount of milk in each bottle and offer smaller but more frequent feeds.

Once feeding challenges have been ruled out, your doctor might want to do a trial of medication for a month to see if their symptoms improve and if they return once the medicine is stopped. Sometimes, we think medication is helping, but things got better because the baby grew out of it.

(Information in this section was taken from the NICE guidance: *Gastro-oesophageal reflux disease in children and young people: diagnosis and management* (NICE, 2019).

It's CMPA

When babies are fussy, some practitioners suggest that it's a cows' milk protein allergy (CMPA).

Cows' milk has a protein that isn't naturally in human milk. These proteins can pass into human milk when Mum consumes milk, cheese, yogurt, or ice cream. Babies' reactions can include:

- Excessive crying
- Eczema
- A sniffly nose that doesn't clear up
- Blood or mucus in poo

They might have a bit of dry skin, which is often dismissed as due to central heating or washing powder. Sometimes, practitioners suggest that parents eliminate dairy products from their diet if their babies are cluster feeding or exhibiting other normal (but challenging) baby behaviour.

While some babies are allergic to cows' milk protein, we need to be careful about overdiagnosing it because it requires the mum to eliminate dairy from her diet, often a big ask when adjusting to life with a new baby. While this isn't a problem for some parents, others would find a complete dietary change to be challenging, and so it doesn't seem fair to suggest a dairy-free diet to a mother without good reason to do so.

As with all things infant feeding related, we need to rule out problems with latching, milk supply, or overfeeding with a bottle before we jump into something bigger.

It's Not CMPA

On the other hand, true cases of CMPA are often dismissed. Ideally, we would have a system where dieticians and IBCLCs work together in cases like this, but in the UK, you'd be incredibly lucky to see either, never mind both. I remember sitting in my GPs office, asking if I should consider cutting dairy from my diet for my baby, who was either asleep or screaming. He had eczema and was forever snotty. My GP said that dairy elimination was a fad and that if my son had CMPA, he would have blood in his stool and be unwell. As a result, it wasn't until he broke out in hives 2 months later when we started solids that we were able to recognise his allergy and adjust my diet accordingly. If latching or other issues have genuinely been ruled out, then CMPA is one possibility to e explore.

Your Baby Is Lactose Intolerant

Newsflash: human milk contains lactose. Human babies are supposed to consume it. Having said that, a few babies each year are born with a true lactose allergy called galactosemia. If a baby has galactosemia, you will know about it quicky. The symptoms are serious and often noticed in the first few days of life. Babies may be allergic to something that's gotten into their mum's milk from her diet, but it would be incredibly rare for them to be allergic to an ingredient that is supposed to be there, like lactose.

Put Them Down Drowsy but Awake

This comes from the idea that babies need to self soothe. Many think that if babies go into their cot while awake, they will learn to fall asleep without being held. This might work for some babies, but we're forgetting that human milk contains hormones that makes them sleep. Falling asleep at the breast is normal behaviour. Think about it from an evolutionary standpoint; if babies are held, they are safe from sabre-toothed tigers. If they are left alone, they could get eaten. It makes sense that human milk, and the act of sucking, makes babies feel safe, relaxed, and sleepy. Westerners fear "making a rod for your own back" or "creating bad sleep habits." However, around the world and throughout most of history, babies have fallen asleep in arms. Babies will learn to sleep on their own when the time is right. Parents shouldn't be made to feel like they're doing something wrong when they feed their little ones to sleep for a few weeks, months, or even years. Perhaps, just make sure your bladder is empty before you settle in for a long bedtime feed.

Bedsharing Will Lead to Sudden Infant Death Syndrome

We used to have a blanket ban on talking about bedsharing, as public health officials feared that talking to parents about would increase the rate of SIDS. However, in recent years, we have learned that SIDS happens when certain safety criteria are not met. In the UK, we now take a different approach. We talk to parents about the risk of *unplanned* bedsharing. This change happened because researchers found that SIDS often occurred when babies and parents fell asleep while on a sofa or in an armchair; if the parent had alcohol, medication, or other substances in their system; the room was too hot; either parent smokes; the baby was sleeping on their stomach, or was premature or poorly. Breastfeeding lowers SIDS rates, even when only partial. Because of these findings, we now talk about the La Leche League Safe Sleep 7. Bedsharing is safe when parents adhere to all these rules.

1. Babies on their backs
2. Not overdressed/swaddled/covered with blankets
3. Everyone in the bed is sober (drugs, alcohol, sedating medication)
4. No one in the bed is a smoker

5. Baby was born full term and is currently healthy
6. Baby is exclusively breastfed
7. The bed is firm, and all pillows and blankets are out of the way.

Oversupply Is a Good Thing

I hear this all the time: "I wish I had an oversupply" or "Surely, giving myself an oversupply by pumping is better than having low supply?" Given our society's obsession with low milk supply and the pervasive idea that women cannot make enough milk to feed their babies, I am not surprised that mothers would think an oversupply seems desirable. We want to be sure that our babies are getting enough milk, so encouraging our bodies to make extra seems logical. Unfortunately, the difficulties oversupply cause are not small inconveniences. I have supported more than a few mums who have ended up in hospital having abscesses drained due to having too much milk.

Unfortunately, there can be too much of a good thing. Let's first consider the symptoms of an overabundant milk supply:

- A baby that chokes, splutters, and gags on the breast
- A baby that is unwilling to latch
- A baby who becomes distressed at the breast
- Blocked milk ducts
- Mastitis
- Breast abscess
- Explosive green nappies, many times a day, often causing nappy rash
- Clothing and bedding being soaked through often, necessitating many changes of clothes and sleeping on piles of towels

- Embarrassment about breastfeeding in public due to the risk of the baby pulling off on let-down, or clothes being soaked
- Difficulties with reducing or ending breastfeeding due to increased risk of breast infections

In short, oversupply is miserable! Excessive pumping can cause oversupply. Some parents are prone to what I call, "All the Milk!"

Luckily, there are things we can do to make this easier for both the parent and baby. First, consider that an oversupply is common in the first few weeks after your baby arrives: your body doesn't know if you've had one baby, two, or three. So, it makes lots of milk just to be sure everyone is fed. Once it figures out how much milk is needed, supply tends to settle for most mums, usually somewhere around week six.

If you're still having trouble with the symptoms I listed above, and it's been longer than 6 weeks, talk to a breastfeeding supporter about reducing supply by only offering one breast per feed or, if things are difficult, block feeding.

CHAPTER 5

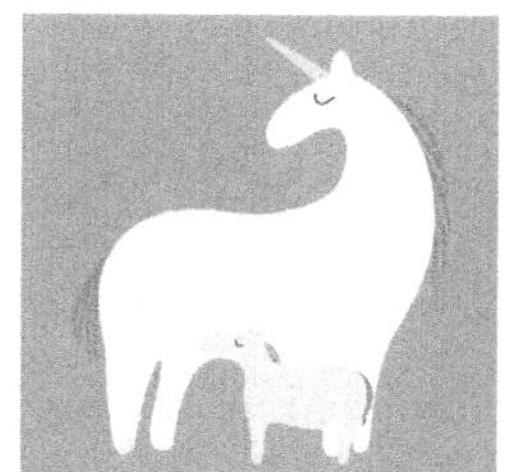

Breastfeeding Your Older Baby

You've survived the first weeks and months of parenting and human milk feeding. Congratulations! Hopefully, the drama is all behind you. If it's not, then please seek support

Introducing Solids Reduces Breastfeeds

I remember standing at the sink and mugs at a breastfeeding group I volunteered for. A friend appeared with my 7-month-old who was happily playing on the floor. She said, "I think he wants boob." I sighed and replied with a laugh, "I thought they're meant to feed less when we give them food, not more!" There began a conversation with all the mothers whose babies were older than six months. They all shared how their babies loved what we called a "boob chaser" with every meal. After a "boob starter" too.

When starting out, solids are like play for most babies. Yes, they need the nutrients available in food, but not a whole lot. More than anything, eating teaches them about texture, hand-eye coordination, and marks the beginning of their lifelong relationship with food. Breastmilk still makes up a huge amount of their daily intake. Even when they are 12 months old, many babies don't seem to eat many solids but are nonetheless chunky, happy, little souls meeting all of their developmental milestones.

We also need to remember that breastmilk isn't simply about nutrition for little ones. It's so much more. Babies may get tired from exploring food and seek the breast to relax and rest. They may need some milk to wash down their meal and want to breastfeed after eating because, why not?

Some babies reduce breastfeeds quite quickly after taking to solids, though this could be because parents give more solids, and spoon-feeding easily fills a tummy leaving no room for milk. Use your baby's hunger and full cues to guide you, and ensure that the breast is always available to them. Some little ones won't "ask" for a feed at this age but will happily take some milk if it's offered.

For a lot more depth on weaning, I recommend Amy Brown's *Why Starting Solids Matters*, and Gill Rapley's book, *Baby-Led Weaning*.

Food Is Only for Fun Until They're 1

While there is quite a lot of truth to this statement, it isn't quite that simple. While human milk provides babies" nutritional needs for the first year, we need to be mindful of our babies' diet from around 6 months. Babies are born with their own store of iron, but this begins to run out at about 6 months. Human milk isn't high in iron, but the iron in breastmilk is well absorbed by babies. Zinc is also not a big ingredient in a mum's milk. After 6 months, babies need food as sources of iron and zinc. This isn't something to be worried about, though; offering food in steadily increasing amounts, as most weaning advice will tell you, alongside continued responsive breastfeeding will usually see that your baby gets everything they need. However, we are offering food for a little bit more than fun and exploration.

You Need to Stop Breastfeeding by 12 Months

Many mammals will nurse their young beyond a year, including cows, elephants, and bears. Our closest cousins, chimps, breastfeed for about 5 years, with gorillas feeding their young for around 4 years.

History also reveals humans breastfed longer than is currently fashionable. In the Medieval period, women in parts of Britain breastfed for at least 18 months, and the ancient Romans and Greeks were keen that children be breastfed into their 3rd year.

Currently, the World Health Organisation recommends that children breastfeed for 2 years and beyond. Many national health organisations make similar recommendations. They based these recommendations on: The human immune system, oral development, and the norm in countries and societies not influenced by formula milk.

The World Health Organisation Guidance About 2 Years and Beyond Is Only for Developing Countries

People assume that WHO refer only to countries outside of the West, but they're not. The recommendation to feed for at least 2 years is for all children and mothers. Here is their statement:

> WHO and UNICEF recommend that children initiate breastfeeding within the first hour of birth and be exclusively breastfed for the first 6 months of life—meaning no other foods or liquids are provided, including water.
>
> Infants should be breastfed on demand—that is as often as the child wants, day and night. No bottles, teats or pacifiers should be used.
>
> From the age of 6 months, children should begin eating safe and adequate complementary foods while continuing to breastfeed for up to 2 years and beyond.

There is no mention of this only being the case for some locations. WHO have also created the Global Breastfeeding Collective (the clue is in the name) and have a *global* monitoring network to ensure that breastmilk substitutes are not unethically marketed.

Your Baby Needs a Routine

Routine is a tricky word. It implies that things stay the same day in, day out, for months or years. Babies, however, tend to change their needs suddenly and often. Perhaps you bring your new baby home, and you find that in the first week, your baby always wakes for a 2-am feed, so you decide to build a routine around that. One week later, your baby wakes at midnight and 4 am as well. Is the routine the problem? No. Your baby just doesn't have any regard for schedules. Babies are hungry when they are hungry, and tired when they are tired. This will change *a lot* in the first 2 years of their life.

It be might helpful to think about patterns, though. For example, as babies get older, they might be ready for a nap about 2 hours after waking up. You can use this as a rough guide for timing naps/feeds/trips to the shops. When babies wake up, you can change their nappies. That's another part of your daily pattern sorted. After a nappy change, your baby may want to feed, have a look around, coo, and pull your hair. There's your morning routine sorted without any pesky clocks getting in the way. Because you're not tied to a schedule that says that your baby needs to wake up at 7:02 am and feed for 16 minutes, you are free to change things.

You Can't Carry on If You Go Back to Work

I think this might be more of a concern in the UK than in places like the U. S., because in Britain, we usually take close to 12 months of maternity leave, while our sisters in America return to work before their babies are 3 months old. In the States, moms to take pumping breaks and their babies to be bottle-fed breastmilk while they work. Here in the UK, pump breaks are far less common, partly because of our maternity leave, but also because so many mothers have stopped breastfeeding before returning to work.

However, those still breastfeeding when they return to work are often told to stop so that they don't have to interrupt their workday to express milk. This simply is not true.

If you return to work when your baby is 12 months old, they are likely to be happy with solid food and water while you are away. You can breastfeed when you are together in the evenings, on weekends, and overnight. Your breasts are less likely to become uncomfortably full at this stage, but you are within your rights, under UK law, to express if you need to.

If you are returning to work and your baby is exclusively breastmilk fed, then it is still possible that your baby can continue to receive your milk (if you want to, of course). You'll need to pump regularly (about every 3 hours, so 2 or 3 times in an average working day, depending on commute), or have your baby brought to you for feedings. You could, of course, do a combination of the two.

> *Lots of people wondered how I'd go back to work while kids were still feeding and without giving formula. I went back to work around 1 year with first child and 8 months with second child, including international travel and both fed till they self-weaned at age 3 for first child and 4.5 for the second child.* ◆ **Madhu**

Teeth Are Problematic

People may tell you that you should stop breastfeeding once your baby has teeth. The logic here is usually that the baby could now bite you. As many mothers know, babies can bite long before they have teeth.

If babies are latched properly, they can't bite you. Because their tongue covers their bottom teeth, preventing them from clamping down.

Some babies go through a biting stage as their teeth come through. Fortunately, this stage is usually short-lived and happens towards the end of a breastfeed, when the flow is slowing down. We can resolve this by either taking the baby off as soon as we feel the subtle shift in latch that often comes before a bite or trying breast compressions to keep the flow of milk fast enough to hold the baby's interest. Teethers can also soothe their gums.

Toddlers do often leave little teeth dents in Mum's breast, typically with the top teeth. This doesn't usually hurt, but if it does, matters can be improved by reattaching the nursling so they are tucked in closer to Mum, in an exaggerated nose-to-nipple position. For older babies, you can even open your mouth wide to encourage them to latch with that nice, wide gape.

Breastmilk Is No Longer Important

Breastmilk is amazing. Some of the immunological factors become more concentrated as the baby gets older and is exposed to more bacteria through crawling, solid foods, and adventuring further away from Mama. Keep in mind that the human immune system isn't fully developed until age 6. Breastmilk's ability to increase its protective factors is useful.

Breastmilk also helps if your little one is poorly and doesn't want to eat solid foods or drink water. They will often still breastfeed instead, and will gain a significant portion of their typical daily micronutrient and macronutrient needs. This can lead to less chances of your toddler being admitted to hospital with dehydration.

On a similar note, breastmilk is often better tolerated than plain water if a child has a vomiting bug. It's softer on the tummy and quickly absorbed, meaning that even if little one is sick soon after, some milk already had the chance to hydrate and soothe.

> *My GP told me, at 14-weeks postnatal, that I needed to give up breast-feeding, as it had no nutritional benefit after 12 weeks. He said his wife was a paediatrician, so he knew what he was talking about. Thankfully, I ignored him and carried on for 12 months.* ◆ Claire

When You Stop Breastfeeding, Your Baby Loses All the Protection Anyway

This bizarre argument is that mothers waste their time by breastfeeding past a certain age. "What does it matter anyway? They'll soon pick up stomach bugs when they wean like every other child."

Apart from the odd logic of wanting to stop a protection sooner because it won't last, many benefits of breastmilk do remain after weaning, including:

- Protection against gastroenteritis for 7 years if you breastfeed for 13 weeks (Howie, 1990).
- Protection against ear infections for 3 years if you breastfeed for four months (Duncan et al., 1993).
- Protection against respiratory infections for 6 to7 years when you breastfeed for 15 weeks (Wilson et al., 1998).
- Protection against Hodgkin's disease when you breastfeed for 6 months, but we're not sure how long that protection lasts (Davis, 1998).

If Your Period Returns, You Need to Stop Breastfeeding

I'm not sure where this one comes from. Lots of women find their milk supply temporarily reduces in the few days around the start of their cycle each month. This, alongside hormonal changes, may change milk's taste, but breastfeeding does not need to end. Babies who rely on breastmilk typically nurse more often if supply is reduced around Mum's period, getting their needs met with more feeds. Once a new cycle begins, milk returns within a few days. Some parents find that magnesium and vitamin C supplements help minimise the effects of period-induced low milk supply.

Exclusive Breastfeeding Will Stop Your Periods Returning

Exclusive breastfeeding can certainly delay your periods returning, but there is no guarantee. It depends on how often a baby is feeding. Frequent overnight feeds delay the return of menstruation further. Regardless, some women do get their periods back after 6 weeks, despite exclusive breastfeeding. We also don't really know if long breastfeeding delays periods returning, as it seems to depend on different lifestyles.

Studies also find it hard to pinpoint what mums can expect regarding their first postnatal period while they're still breastfeeding. One found that some women could breastfeed 15 times a day and still get their periods back before their baby's 6-month birthday (Elias et al., 1986).

A safe suggestion for when to expect a first period (and the return of fertility) is around 6 months The baby nurses less with the introduction of solids so the menstrual cycle is more likely to start again. Some mums, however, may find that their periods don't return for a year or more, if they continue breastfeeding.

A method of contraception called the Lactational Amenorrhea Method (LAM) can work well, as long as:

- The baby is under 6 months of age.
- The baby is exclusively breastfed, with no supplements.
- The baby feeds around the clock.
- Mum doesn't have her period back yet.

However, while this method is about 98% protective against pregnancy, it does not protect against STDs (Fabic & Choi, 2013) and should stop being relied upon as soon as even one of the criteria ceases happening.

> *"You can't get pregnant whilst breastfeeding." Erm... Yes, yes, I did. She's now 13 months and tandem feeding alongside her 4½-year-old sister.* ◆ **Shell**

CHAPTER 6

Toddlerhood and Beyond: why Natural Term Breastfeeding Isn't Weird

Of all breastfeeding topics, the most controversial is breastfeeding after babyhood. In the UK, this appears to be an issue sometime after the baby turns a year old. Formula feeding has influenced our thinking when it's time to stop breastfeeding. Unfortunately, these beliefs contradict both history and biology. In this chapter, I'll discuss the myths around breastfeeding toddlers that will give you the confidence to ignore people who think breastmilk for a 2-year-old is odd.

Before we dive in, it seems like a sensible idea to explore global recommendations for breastfeeding:

- The World Health Organisation: 2 years and beyond
- The CDC in the USA: 12 months
- The NHS: 2nd year and beyond
- National Health and Medical Research Council in Australia: 12 to 24 months
- Ministry of Health (New Zealand): At least 1 year
- The German National Breastfeeding Committee: As long as the Mother and Child wish

- In Islam: Two lunar years (about 22 days before the baby turns 2)
- Buddhism (historically): 6 to7 years
- Average natural term weaning age globally: Age 4 (range 3 to 7 yrs)

Do please bear the above in mind as we now enter the murky waters of "Well, I just think it's weird."

Now Your Baby Can Walk, They Don't Need Breastmilk

People put random limitations on breastfeeding duration. These are bizarre when you understand that human milk is so much more than calories and vitamins. A walking toddler may want to breastfeed more often than a 4- or 5-month-old. They are exploring the world with new freedom, and that can be both exciting and scary. What could be more logical than to check in with Mum for a quick feed before toddling off to explore some more? Lysozyme becomes more concentrated in toddlers' breastmilk because, as they are more exposed to different toys, sticks, play equipment at the park, and climbing all over the dog, they are picking up more bacteria. Lysozyme's job is to eat bacteria, and that is one of my favourite breastmilk facts.

If They Can Ask for It, It's Weird

People seem to forget (or not realise) that a newborn asks for milk. This is what hunger cues are for, and it's why we teach parents to be aware of them. A 5-month-old will nuzzle into mum's chest when it's time to feed, therefore, asking for milk. I taught my babies to sign. My eldest was a keen learner and could sign "milk" by 7 months old.

Of course, I know what people are talking about when they say, "Babies are too old now that they can ask for it," is the ability to verbally request a feed. People feel uncomfortable when a 3-year-old says they want "boob," "milkies," or "mummy milk," because breasts are sexualised. If you ask people why a child asking to breastfeed is weird, they often say things like, "they're too old" or "it's just weird to hear that." Even "I don't want to know about it; it's private." Someone needs to ask these people how they feel when a 3-year-old declares to an entire room that they need to do a poo, which is also something that people don't want to hear about. I'm not equating breastfeeding to bowel movements here; it's just odd what people decide is okay and what is not okay.

If They Can Help Themselves, it's Inappropriate

Much the same as the above section, newborns can help themselves. All you need to do is put them on your bare tummy and they will use their reflexes to wriggle up to the breast and latch on. We should all be able to help ourselves to the comfort and nutrition we need. Why on Earth should breastfeeding be any different? Comfort is a wonderful thing to be able to seek and should surely be encouraged.

Of course, a second argument here is about boundaries and bodily autonomy. Toddlers and little ones pulling at your clothes, or exposing your body when you don't want them to, is absolutely something you can stop. It's totally okay to have boundaries here. It's your body, after all.

Stopping Will Make Them Sleep Better

I'd love to promise you more sleep. Unfortunately, ending breastfeeding will likely not do that for you. In fact, many mothers find that when breastfeeding ends, they lose the only tool they have for maximising time spent in the land of dreams.

Toddlers wake at night for many reasons: because they are cold, hot, thirsty, uncomfortable, they have an itch, they're scared, lonely, or because it's a day that ends in a Y. While it's true that, for some toddlers, reducing or stopping night feeds seems to help them sleep longer, there is absolutely no guarantee that this will be the case for *your* little one.

Make sure that your pre-bedtime and bedtime routines are spotless, and you may want to see if rooming in with your toddler makes wakeups happen more or less often, or has no impact at all. Checking that naps are optimal also helps when toddlers are waking lots at night.

You could also try layering up some extra sleepy cues, such as ambient noise, essential oils, and/or a nightlight projector that displays stars or animals on the ceiling. Avoid blue light, from screens, such cell phones and e-readers, because it tells your brain that you're awake.

If you have perfected all of the above for sleep hygiene, then you might want to think about some gentle nudges towards night weaning. There are some amazing books to help you with that, such as *A Loving Weaning*, or you could talk to an IBCLC.

You Can't Have a Sex Life

Anyone that thinks stopping breastfeeding will somehow free up more time for sex is deluded, frankly. Anyone that views their need for sex above their children's needs should re-evaluate their attitude towards the mother of their baby.

You Won't Want a Sex Life

Fortunately, most women don't feel that breastfeeding has a big negative impact on their sex lives in the long run. Avery, Duckett, and Frantzich (2000) asked 576 American women about this, and the mothers concluded that there was a small negative impact, with 60% saying this was primarily around breast stimulation during sex.

Sperm Will Contaminate Your Milk

This myth, first recorded in Medieval England, is about a strange theory that the uterus and breast are connected, and that semen contaminates milk by its contact with the uterus. Maher (1992) concluded that this myth was strong enough to cause early cessation of breastfeeding. Happily, though, there is no connection between the breast and uterus, which is one reason why fertility issues don't lead to breastfeeding issues.

It's Just for Mum

First of all, so what? Personally, I'll happily take a reduction in breast cancer risks as a result of breastfeeding, thank you very much (Anstey et al., 2017). On this topic, here's a fascinating fact for you; in 1977, Ing et al. looked at women breastfeeding in the fishing villages in Hong Kong. Traditionally, these mothers only breastfed from the right breast. The study found a fourfold increased risk of breast cancer in the mums' left breasts. Feel free to share that one next time someone claims someone is *still* breastfeeding for selfish reasons.

There are other benefits to mothers and are great examples of why breastfeeding for yourself is a perfectly valid reason to carry on.

- A 4% to 12% reduced risk for type 2 diabetes for every 12 months of lactation.
- A 28% reduction in the risk of ovarian cancer if you breastfeed for 12 months.
- Delayed return of periods (which, for some women, continues for the duration of breastfeeding, even into years), which saves money on menstrual products, eliminates PMS symptoms, and provides natural child spacing.
- Reduced risk of heart disease during and after lactation.
- A closer bond with their children.
- Easier weight loss due to the additional calories burned, even in late lactation. (Dieterich et al., 2012).

Secondly, parents breastfeed children for longer than the societal norm of 12 or 24 months because they can see how happy it makes their child, and it reassures them regarding their children's immune system and all the bugs small kids pick up. They don't do it for themselves.

Breastfeeding a toddler or an older little one is not a walk in the park. If you spend 24 with a breastfed toddler and their parent, you will observe the child requesting milk, endlessly, and often, Mum saying, "not right now," or words to the same effect. Other challenges include poor latch, aversion, feeling exhausted, and societal pressures to stop.

> *(I was told) That I shouldn't breastfeed once she was a year old, as there was no benefit to her, and it was just for me. [It was] Disproved by using my local resources and antenatal information, as well as the WHO organisation. Also, anyone who thought it was just for me was clearly delusional! I loved feeding my wee girl, but it was hard a lot of the time too.* ◆ **Nic**

It Will Cause Problems Once They Start School

> *I was told that she'll be too clingy and won't settle when she starts school, she'll just ask for boobies.* ◆ **Jade**

For some reason, people imagine that if children are still breastfeeding when they start school, their mother is going to be standing at the playground fence, poking a boob through for her little one at lunchtime.

Breastfeeding a school-age child is nothing like that. It's usually a feed in the morning before school, and a feed or three after school (typically at home). Breastmilk is not used instead of solid food, and the child is probably used to going to daycare without breastfeeding, anyway.

The other argument is that children will be teased. My answer is twofold. Firstly, how will anyone know the child is breastfed? Typically, mums are fed up with being shamed in public. By the time their child is 4, they only feed at home. Children are highly unlikely to be going to school and telling all their friends about breastfeeding because it is so normal to them. It's like getting a drink of water or a cuddle—it is a given.

Secondly, if children tease others about breastfeeding, they have to have learned somewhere. Four- and 5-year-olds don't bat an eyelid at their peers breastfeeding unless someone has told them it's weird. So, adults who worrying about teasing may want to consider where children are getting these ideas.

My 4.5-year-old has just started reception and at her parent's evening, we were told she's like a mother to the children and goes over to anyone who looks sad and plays with everyone. ◆ **Jade**

Night Feeds Cause Tooth Decay

Night feeds are unlikely to cause tooth decay as long as you brush children's teeth twice a day. When a toddler is breastfeeding, milk bypasses the teeth and goes straight down their throats. Breastmilk also contains lactoferrin, an ingredient that destroys the bacteria most likely to cause caries.

A 1990 study in Finland found no link between breastfeeding and caries up to 3 years of age (Alaluusua, 1990). Another study stated that "human breast milk in not cariogenic" (Erickson, 1999).

Research into human skulls from 500 to 1,000 years ago found that cavities were historically rare. People were predominantly breastfed, possibly for a long time. This suggests that breastfeeding did not cause dental caries.

Unfortunately, many dentists argue that teeth don't know the difference between breastmilk sugar and any other types, and that they see exclusively breastfed toddlers in their practices who have cavities. One school of thought suggests that cavities may be due to little ones falling asleep with milk in their mouths. However, this is not an issue with breastfed children, as milk stops flowing once they are no longer sucking.

Genes may also be at play here, but we're not sure. Common-sense advice is to brush teeth well, twice a day, and make sure your little one has regular dental check-ups. Limit or avoid artificial teats in older babies and toddlers, including dummies, and monitor sugar intake in their diet.

It's Sexual

I don't even want to call this one a myth. It's a disgusting, ignorant accusation that demonstrates perfectly the issues some people have with breasts. Luckily, most people no longer hold this view. Unfortunately, the older the nursling is, the more likely that some vile internet troll will claim the mother is getting sexual gratification from her child being at the breast. Some mums say that the nipple stimulation (often from a shallow latch) can lead to feelings of arousal, but these feelings are not linked to the act of feeding; just the stimulation. Mums who are brave enough to share these feelings are often ashamed and worried something is wrong with them and want to stop breastfeeding, even though the arousal is in no way linked to their baby or breastfeeding itself (Mueller, 1985).

No One Wants to See THAT

The person making this comment probably doesn't want to see you breastfeeding because they are so uncomfortable with the female body. It takes a special type of person to assume their opinions are widely held. I don't particularly want to see Piers Morgan on my TV, but for some reason, millions of people seem to like him, so I just change the channel when he pops up. I don't want him banned from our screens just because I don't like him.

There is, of course, a much bigger issue here. We're back to breasts being primarily sexual. I recently had a frustrating discussion with a parent and baby group. They decided that since babies unlatched and left their mothers "exposed" that breastfeeding should not happen in their setting. They claimed that they were safeguarding mothers since there were men in the room. They also argued that this wasn't a breastfeeding issue since babies weren't feeding when they were unlatched. The issue was female exposure. Numerous people cited the law protecting breastfeeding in public. Despite this, the group upheld their policy that breastfeeding was private to protect the mum and baby. The undertone was clear; your breasts are sexual, and a man might be turned on by a flash of your nipple.

There is so much I could say about this topic, not least that our view of breasts as sexual is nothing more than cultural nonsense. If someone is looking hard enough to see a nipple, we should ask them why they're staring. The baby has every right to pause and move away from the breast before going back to their feed, without it being implied that the parent is exposing herself. All of this goes away if we don't live in a society that sexualises milk-making tissue.

"If You Can Breastfeed in public, Why Can't I Urinate in Public?"

This retort is another social media favourite you don't hear in your local coffee shop or over dinner, but it's out there. The argument is that breastmilk is a bodily fluid, like urine, so why can't a man just whip out his penis and pee in the street?

My favourite response is, "Do you *want* to pee in the street?" or "Are you saying you want to feed a baby your urine?"

I mean, come on. This argument isn't even worth pulling apart because it's so ridiculous (and clearly designed to shock and provoke a reaction, not a genuine concern people have). Toilets exist for bowel and bladder needs, not for baby-feeding. You can eat in the street, whether you are a baby or an adult. Urine is full of bacteria while breastmilk is full of antibodies. Breastfeeding in public is protected by law while public urination is absolutely not.

"How Would You Feel If We Just Let Men Wave Their Willies Around?"

Someone actually said this to me. Alarmingly, it was used as a legitimate reason for why mothers couldn't breastfeed their babies at a public meeting. First of all, penises are primarily sexual organs while breasts are not. Secondly, a waste product is eliminated through a penis, whereas nutrition is secreted by breasts. Thirdly, breastfeeding is public is protected by the law, while "waving your willy around" in public is deemed indecent exposure.

"You're making your child a Mummy's boy"

Some believe that breastfed older baby or toddler is clingier" towards the lactating parent. Rather than celebrating a secure emotional attachment, our Western world sees this as a problem. Parents are told that they have created a "Mummy's boy," with the idea that children are unable to socialise because they lack confidence or independence. Hundreds of studies have found the opposite to be true. For example, one review found:

> Heightened socio-affective responding seen in breastfed children is possibly connected to the stimulation of the oxytocin system and oxytocin's known role in promoting positive affect and approach behaviors, while reducing stress and avoidance behavior (Krol & Grossmann, 2018).

In other words, breastfeeding children seem happier, less stressed, and they pay more attention to positive cues from people around them (such as smiling/softened eyes). This study suggests that oxytocin is at work.

Another study looked at the breastfeeding practices for 999 mother-infant pairs. A group of children, aged 15 to 18 years, were assessed using several psychosocial measures, including parent/child relationships, juvenile delinquency, substance abuse, and mental health. The children who were breastfed for longer than 4 months were more likely to describe their mothers as more caring and less overprotective compared to their bottle-fed friends. The authors concluded that extended breastfeeding did not increase the risk of mental health problems, but breastfeeding can result in closer parent/child relationships. This means that while breastfeeding children seem to grow closer to their mothers, that relationship doesn't have a negative effect on them (Horwood & Fergusson, 1998).

Consistent with Horwood and Fergusson's (1998) findings, many other studies found that baby/parent bonding leads to better social skills later on. So, if breastfeeding increases bonding, and bonding leads to stronger social skills, we can be confident that being a "Mummy's boy" is not a problem. In fact, Joas and Mohler (2021) sum it up well:

> The present data confirm a positive and long-term influence of bonding on social skills and provide further evidence of the importance of parent-child bonding for child development in general.

CHAPTER 7

Pregnancy and Tandem Feeding

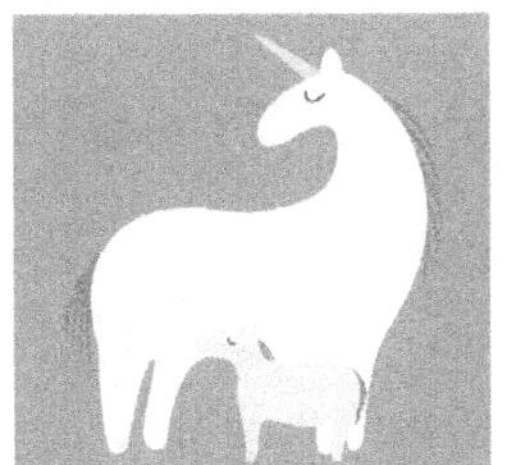

There are many myths around breastfeeding through pregnancy and then tandem feeding children of different ages. One part of the problem is that many mothers aren't breastfeeding long enough to think about whether it's safe to continue in pregnancy. If they do, they typically don't talk about it outside of their inner circle of breastfeeding friends and supporters. Unfortunately, that prevents it from ever becoming a talking point in the wider community.

Breastfeeding In Pregnancy Causes Miscarriage

Many believe that oxytocin released while breastfeeding stimulates contractions and increases the risk of miscarriage. Thankfully, this is unlikely to happen until the end of pregnancy. Progesterone, which is present in large amounts during pregnancy, blocks the uterus from surges in oxytocin (Flower, 2003). The only caution I want to give is that if you have a history of preterm labour, you might want to avoid breastfeeding in pregnancy. If your body is gearing up for another early labour, those oxytocin surges might be allowed to interact with your uterus, potentially tipping you over into another premature labour. There's limited research on this, but it feels like a sensible precaution.

Your Toddler Will Wean

Your toddler might wean, or they might not. We can't say for sure which way things will go. For many mothers, their milk supply reduces significantly during pregnancy. While some toddlers don't mind this, others will stop nursing if supply is dwindling. If you want to tandem feed, it can help to keep your breast available to your little one for comfort as well as nourishment. Toddlers who nurse for comfort are more likely to continue feeding through pregnancy than the toddler who feeds only for the milk.

Your Toddler Will Take Colostrum Away from Your Newborn

Colostrum is only available for a few days after your baby is born. In most cases, newborns and their mothers spend a lot of time together and do a lot of feeding, while the older sibling is likely in daycare or spending time with loved ones. We want to make sure that newborns have plenty of opportunity to take colostrum, as it's so important for their tiny guts. However, there is no real reason to stop your older child from feeding as well. Mohrbacher (2010) suggests giving your newborn priority at the breast to ensure that they get lots of colostrum. The older child can feed afterwards, a few times a day. This might even help to prevent engorgement as milk begins to become more abundant around day 3. Georgie shares her personal experience of tandem feeding her newborn and toddler:

> My daughter was 2.5 when my son was born, and I was so worried that my supply would be affected during my pregnancy, as she breastfed many times a day, although she had stopped at night. It was so lovely having milky snuggles during my pregnancy and I took photos each month of the bump and usually, she was latched too! Around month 8, I started getting aversion and that began 6 months of horrific feelings, where I adored her but wanted to throw her across the room rather than feed, so we developed a "latch for

one song duration" habit. It took another year to go completely, and she had her last feed when she was around 5.

When my son was born, she breastfed before he even did, and tandem feeding began. It surprised me how strong his latch was compared to hers. I thought it wouldn't be much different. I would feed them both when she wanted to. Sometimes, they'd both have both sides and sometimes, it was just one of them. I'd feed them to sleep together, and we'd nap together in the afternoon, which was bliss. Breastfeeding was an enormous part of her life, and I was happy that she wouldn't lose this precious time.

I was aware that I might need to offer to the baby first, and thought I'd just see how it went. I did consciously offer one side to him first if the eldest wanted some, to make sure he got the milk he needed. That lasted a couple of weeks, at most. But no sticking to one side, no conscious 'he had that side last time so needs to have this side now.'

Tillie shares her experience, with a great example of how nipple stimulation from breastfeeding doesn't lead to early labour:

I fell pregnant with my youngest daughter whilst still breastfeeding her older sister. Beatrix was 2 at the time and showed no signs of slowing or stopping. I had some sensitivity in the early stages of my pregnancy, so I really had to be cautious with her latch. At around 14 weeks, I realised the sensation had changed and when I checked, by hand expressing, I realised that my milk had completely dried up. Beatrix continued nursing throughout my pregnancy and seemed to have no problems with dry nursing. She still fed as much as previously, although she did naturally night wean at this point, so although she still fed to sleep, she didn't feed overnight. At around 28 weeks, my colostrum returned, it was plentiful, and Beatrix certainly wasn't expecting it the night it came back but she was happy to be getting milk once again.

Once baby was born (at a very tardy 43+2 so the feeding did not cause early contractions/labour for me), I tandem fed Beatrix, who was now 3, and my newborn, Ophelia. My colostrum changed very quickly to a great milk supply, and they would often feed together, holding hands, or stroking each other's hair and face. They're now 5 and 2, and both still feeding, though Beatrix only feeds every few days now, but it's been a lovely, natural progression to get to where we are, and I definitely feel that continuing to feed Beatrix throughout pregnancy and after having Ophelia has meant that she still felt connected with me and created a beautiful bond with her sister.

Your Body Won't Make Enough Milk to Tandem Feed

Your body is designed to feed twins and more and exclusively as well. As such, it can certainly handle a newborn and a child on solids. Feeding two children encourages milk production, and your body will respond accordingly, ensuring that both children receive plenty of milk. In fact, it's fairly common for mums to have a degree of oversupply, or a fast let-down when feeding a baby and their older sibling.

It's important to prioritise the baby over the child taking solids foods, so this means offering the baby access to the breast first and making sure they are done with their feed before letting the older child take the milk that is left.

Your Body Will Be Making Toddler Milk

With each birth, our body starts a new lactation. Copious milk supply is triggered by the birth of the placenta, and your body will make milk that prioritises your newborn. Your toddler or older child will also benefit from the availability of extra milk, but this milk will primarily be produced for the baby. A study released in 2021 looked at the milk samples of tandem-feeding mums over 24 hours. They found that milk composition was linked to each child's development, and that all of the babies and children had their nutritional requirements met by their mum's milk (Sinkiewicz-Darol et al., 2021).

Jess shares with us how she breastfed her second baby and her older child together for around a year, after breastfeeding throughout her pregnancy. Contrary to the common myths, breastfeeding certainly didn't result in her baby arriving early, or impact her baby's nutrition after birth:

> I found out I was pregnant days before my son's second birthday, I'd had an extremely difficult start with feeding him, so how this pregnancy would affect our feeding relationship, and how my second breastfeeding journey would go were great concerns to me.
>
> My mother often talked about her own breastfeeding journeys ending due to pregnancy so I had always expected that I would experience something similar. However, my second pregnancy also coincided with a global pandemic. This brought with it fear, uncertainty, and a lot of pyjamas days at home with a toddler.
>
> I was sure I would be happy for my son to wean, and when I experienced some discomfort feeding in the early weeks, it made me even more sure, but he seemed keener than ever and I was grateful for that connection when I felt that sickness, tiredness, and stress was pulling me away from him. So, we took it day by day, week by week. I then considered the discussions about antibodies and the news of the vaccine gave me the idea that I could pass some immunity on to him if I could carry on a little longer.
>
> The discomfort settled after a few weeks and my son seemed happy with the amount of milk I was producing; he would curl up next to me and caress my tummy while he fed, and I would explain about the baby that would be coming soon, that he would be sharing his "milkies" with. Other than the sickness, I had a good pregnancy, all the midwives I met were supportive of my breastfeeding aims, and were unphased by my toddler still feeding. My milk reduced but I don't believe it ever dried up. I was able to collect colostrum easily in the final weeks (in case it was needed for baby), which I hadn't been able to do in my first pregnancy.

I was advised that nipple stimulation would help induce labour, if baby was ready, but no matter how much he fed, my daughter still didn't arrive until I was 13 days overdue. Thankfully, she was an expert feeder from day 1, so my expressed colostrum wasn't needed, and I began a healing process accepting the differences in each baby.

At first, I was nervous of tandem feeding. I would only let my son feed after the baby and for short bursts to "save it" for her. She gained and fed well, so I started to relax on this quite soon. I also learnt to feed them both together and felt like Super Mum, taking them to bed and feeding them both to sleep while they held hands across my middle. My son was extremely affectionate with the baby, and I think feeding together strengthened the bond.

My daughter is 1 tomorrow, she's still an excellent feeder, and usually more interested in milk than food. My son is 4 in a few months, and I think we had our last feed a few weeks ago. I was acutely aware that the last was coming any day, but it tapered off so gently that I'm not sure I could pin it down and there was no sadness or finality on either side.

CHAPTER 8

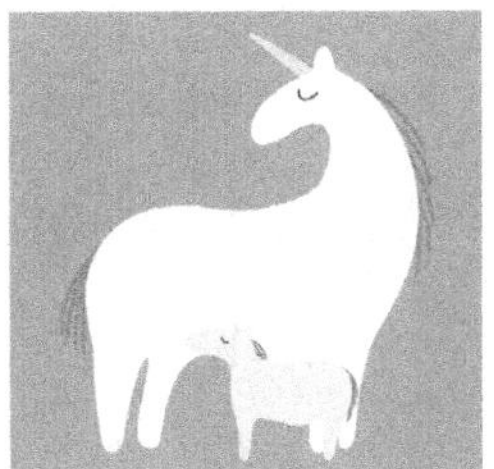

Your Health and Wellbeing

Drugs in Breastmilk

If you see your GP or chemist for a medication and say that you're breastfeeding, they will likely tell you to stop. While a few meds are contraindicated for lactation, most are not. Because of potential legal liability, drug companies tend to issue blanket statements, saying meds are not safe to take if you're breastfeeding. According to the Drugs in Breastmilk Information Service, the following medications are usually safe to take while lactating. This book can't give medical advice, so please check with the Drugs in Breastmilk Information Service or a breastfeeding-friendly GP.

- Off the shelf painkillers, such as paracetamol or ibuprofen (but not codeine or aspirin)
- Hay fever medication (as long as it doesn't contain a decongestant or could make you drowsy)
- Many types of antibiotics
- Cough syrups (non-drowsy and not decongestant types, and as long as no codeine is present)
- Several types of antidepressants
- The progestin-only contraceptive pill (anecdotally, several parents do report reduced milk supply so use with caution)

- Indigestion relief
- Asthma medication
- Insulin
- Warfarin
- Emergency birth control
- Loperamide (for diarrhoea)

Antidepressants

> *I rang my doctors to say I felt like I needed to go back on my antidepressants. The doctor told me I would have to choose between that and breastfeeding. I said that giving up breastfeeding would make me feel even worse, but he essentially said there was no other solution. Thankfully, I have a rather fantastic friend who, after hearing me cry down the phone to her, rang the surgery and gave them an earful. The doctor called me back and admitted he could switch my medication to a different one.* ◆ **Marie**

The Drugs in Breastmilk Information Service has a wonderfully detailed factsheet about antidepressants and breastfeeding. The take-home message is clear: most are safe to take during lactation. Sertraline is most preferred, with Citalopram coming in second, but there are other options as well. I'm so pleased that Marie's friend was able to advocate for her.

Can I Take Paracetamol (Tylenol) at the Same Time as My Baby?

According to the Drugs in Breastmilk Information Service, it is unlikely that enough paracetamol will pass through your milk to be clinically significant, even if your baby is also taking paracetamol. Therefore, they suggest that it is safe for both of you to be taking paracetamol if needed.

Conflicting Information About Codeine

Sometimes, you're told that you can take codeine while breastfeeding, while other times, you might be told that you can't. Current guidance (since 2013) suggests codeine should not be used in lactation, but that other opioids might be safe.

The issue with codeine is that it metabolises into morphine in the body, but the extent of this varies from person to person. Because of this, the side effects are unpredictable, and we don't know who will end up with a lot of morphine in their bloodstream and who won't. If your body is efficient at turning codeine into morphine, your baby will be at increased risk of breathing problems (at least 44 cases of respiratory depression have been reported to the Medicines and Healthcare Products Regulatory Agency), and in 2012, a Canadian baby died at 12 days old because the mother was prescribed codeine (Jones, 2021).

Vegan Breastmilk Is Lacking in Nutrients

The myth that vegan diets are lacking seems to extend to vegan breastmilk. However, there is absolutely no evidence that suggests the baby of a vegan parent won't thrive on human milk alone in the first 6 months of life. The only thing to consider is taking a good vitamin B12 supplement, which many vegans take anyway. Babies do receive this vitamin through Mum's milk, and Mum gets it from her diet. As B12 is primarily found in animal products, it can be hard to get the amount you need from a vegan diet alone, so supplementing is usually needed.

When I asked for experiences from vegan families regarding misinformation and lactation, I received this story from Lilli. It's a little longer than a lot of the accounts here but her story identifies many issues around a lack of knowledge parents can come up against during breastfeeding. She dealt with feeding twins, tandem feeding her older children, allergies, lack of correct information, and poor support, all while defending her right to be vegan.

I had been breastfeeding for 17 months when my second child was born. When he was 4 months old, his behaviours began to change. With my first, I had required IBCLC advice to establish breastfeeding. She gave me so much information to empower me during tongue-tie, slow weight gain, jaundice, blebs, nipple trauma, vasospasms, so when it came to my second child, I felt equipped and actually, with no tongue-tie and brilliant weight gain, had comfortable feeds from the off. I appreciated how different this second experience of breastfeeding was. It also meant the change in his behaviour at 4 months was clear. Something wasn't right. As the weeks went on, he developed the classic symptoms of CMPA. After exhausting all other routes, I looked into nutritional causes of this. I adapted my diet and when it came to weaning and we avoided dairy. The nutritional study became a rabbit hole and led us as a family to going plant based. In the next 18 months, I conceived twins while tandem breastfeeding my baby and toddler. They were 3 and 2 when the twins arrived and were (are) healthy, strong, physically active, and with all milestones accomplished. At this point, I had entered the realm of natural term weaning. With that comes judgment, lack of understanding, and plenty of misinformation.

The twins were born 6 weeks premature. They arrived via vaginal delivery on their own accord. Whisked off to NICU, I was left on postnatal ward, on a mission to express and tube feed. I'd prepared myself for this eventuality and was committed to what it entailed. Basically, very little sleep, ever.

What I hadn't anticipated was the way my choice to keep the twins on breastmilk would be received. I explained to nursing staff how unwell my son was due to dairy in my milk and therefore, I was determined these premature babies would only have my vegan milk (or donor, if required). Building up milk supply and, therefore, increasing a baby's weight takes time. I understood this meant my stay in NICU may have been reduced had I agreed to the use of formula, but I had the long-term health of my children in my mind. There was no medical reason for an alternative milk to be given than to increase their weights faster and clear the incubators. My agenda was to get the twins directly breastfeeding, and when I was correctly supported with this, I was able to release more milk—stress was a huge inhibitor of my milk release.

Phrases and language like "Mum wants to try to breastfeed" became "Mum still wants to try and breastfeed." I was there in the room, with these phrases being spoken over me. The handover staff would glance up at the culprit (me) for this frustrated delay in my milk volume. All the while, not remotely appreciating the milk I was making and the commitment to pumping. It turned out I really only needed an extra 48 hours to express the milk volumes required, and this came as a senior member of staff made it possible for me to stay at the hospital and said my milk would be enough, as the twins weaned off the drips (dextrose), which they'd required since being born. The few who supported me and my wishes (along with friends on my phone) gave me the energy and calm I needed to produce milk. My diet had nothing to do with the amount—this was all inhibited by stress and the strain of having babies in incubators and not on my chest.

As a peer supporter myself, I was aware of language and the lasting effect it can have. It can become the positive or negative earworm during those long newborn nights. Now, I was on the receiving end of witnessing the damage careless language could have. The amount I was having to rely on my own knowledge of breastmilk/breastfeeding and plant-based nutrition was draining. A nursing parent needs lifting and each feed/pump to be celebrated; reassurance is required around the clock.

Weeks down the line, feeding tubes removed, bronchiolitis beaten, breastfeeding exclusively established, I was nursing four children. I then received a letter stating the need to attend an urgent appointment with a paediatric consultant at the hospital. Unbeknownst to me, my health visitor (who hadn't seen us for 5 weeks at this point) had reported concerns about my "vegan" diet affecting the milk quality and the "still" breastfeeding two other children. The consultant looked at both the twins and was embarrassed that I'd had to come to the hospital; they apologised. But I left there with a complete distrust. No concerns had been raised or discussed with me, yet a letter and urgent referral had been sent to my GP and hospital? I had spent so many days and nights doing around the clock feeds and care, I was fragile and exhausted on a level my body hadn't experienced before. To be let down during this time by the professionals I should have been able to turn to was indescribably disappointing.

I declined further health visitor support. I got my own weigh scales. I did a diploma in vegan nutrition and empowered myself further to support the methods, which were working so well for our health as a family.

I am fortunate to have had enough access to informed advice and support, during a time when society has, perhaps, become detached from biological norms.

Statistically, what I achieved with the twins while breastfeeding my older two too is rare in UK culture. Because breastfeeding multiples and to natural term isn't as common, ongoing support is appreciated by the parent. It's a shame to not only not have these achievements celebrated by some medical professionals, but to have it confused as a negative act; this could be so damaging to a parent's health and undermines their instinctual choices. Aside from the effort involved, breast/chest health of the parent and the long-term benefits to the child are sometimes ignored, it felt to me at times like I was the only one fighting for this. I wasn't. I had my own support network, but it's a shame I couldn't turn to the professionals around me during the early years.

Caffeine Will Make Your Baby Jittery

Ah, caffeine, the secret to getting out of bed and the kids to where they need to be on time for many families! You might have heard that you shouldn't consume caffeine if you're breastfeeding, or that you should limit yourself to a conservative amount each day. We know that caffeine can get into breastmilk, and too much of it might lead to a wakeful baby or a baby that's a bit jittery. You probably need to consume quite a lot for this to happen, though. Bear in mind that the older your baby is, the less caffeine seems to bother them, and if solids are well established, they will be taking less milk, and therefore, less caffeine.

Alcohol

Alcohol, like caffeine, seems to have a bit of a bad reputation when it comes to breastfeeding. I remember the horror of a relative of mine when they saw me drinking a bottle of cider (I'm classy) while my baby was latched to my breast. Alcohol consumption during lactation is a little bit tricky to pick apart because there are a few different ideas floating around. Some sources tell you to avoid it altogether, others tell you to stick to two units a day, and some say that if you're sober enough to care for your baby, you're sober enough to breastfeed your baby. It's all confusing, but which is right?

Well, we aren't sure. We're fairly confident some alcohol isn't going to be a problem, as long as you don't then share a sleep space with your baby. We know it leaves your breastmilk as it leaves your blood (so you don't need to pump out alcoholic milk) and we know that most parents don't want to get blind drunk but would like a glass of wine with dinner or a glass of gin.

According to the Drugs and Lactation Database (also known as Lactmed), mothers who regularly drink more than two units of alcohol daily breastfeed for less time than those who don't drink or do so with moderation. It explains that two units daily doesn't seem to cause any short- or long-term problems for babies or parents but cautions that more than five drinks daily can disrupt the milk-ejection reflex (your let-down), making breastfeeding difficult for your baby.

In the same article, Lactmed also tells us that alcohol is present in breastmilk, and the more a mother drinks, the higher those levels are. Babies who are exposed to excessive alcohol consumption via Mum's milk tend to sleep less but more often and are fussy. Some studies found that they temporarily find sucking at the breast hard to coordinate as well. These issues improve as the alcohol leaves Mum's blood, and therefore, her milk.

Long-term exposure to chronic alcohol consumption has been documented as causing slow weight gain and as babies needing hospital admission.

So should you drink while breastfeeding? The answer is much the same as for the general population: drinking occasionally, in moderation (about two units), is unlikely to be problematic for the parent or baby. Each drink takes about 2 hours to clear from your system. Just don't bedshare if there is booze in your system.

Nights Out Are Impossible

It's amazing how rigid people can be when they think about breastfeeding. Feeding a toddler or a child is not the same as feeding a baby solely reliant on human milk. A supportive carer (typically an aunt or grandparent) can help a breastfed toddler to fall asleep either in bed or snuggled up with them on the sofa while parents enjoy a few hours out for dinner or the cinema. If Mum wants to go out with friends, her partner is usually perfectly capable of looking after the little one without the power of the boob for a few hours. Cuddles, snacks, TV—whatever works! Usually, children will fall asleep just a little later than usual, but does it matter if they have an occasional later night? Of course, if your baby is still small, there is no reason to not take them with you to dinner. They will probably just sleep anyway, soothed by the background noise. I wish I'd had the confidence to take my first baby with me to restaurants, wedding receptions, and the cinema when he was tiny.

You Have PND Because You Are Breastfeeding

This myth makes me angry every day. It's a perfect example of how we blame breastfeeding for everything, and breastfeeding is not the problem.

Not meeting your breastfeeding goals and experiencing breastfeeding challenges increase the risk of PND, but breastfeeding that's going well actually protects mothers' mental health.

Women are frequently told to stop breastfeeding if they're depressed. Hormones, tiredness, and stress are typically blamed for their low mood. Yet, many of these mums will say when asked, "But breastfeeding is the one thing I'm enjoying!" Why on Earth do we live in a world where medical professionals think they can tell women what is right for them, despite the mother's own lived experience of the exact opposite? My own experience of the above goes like this:

> My youngest baby, Oliver, didn't feed at the breast. He simply would not do it. So, I pumped for him, and he had my milk in a bottle. I grieved the lack of breastfeeding and was deeply saddened by him not being at my breast, but I was incredibly proud of my exclusive pumping journey, and, in fact, pumping was one constant and consistent thing in my life. I didn't mind it at all; it wasn't something I found particularly challenging, personally.
>
> At my eldest son's 2-year check with the health visitor, she asked me about my mental health. I said I was stressed, tired, and a bit low in mood, but I didn't think I needed treatment. Immediately, the health visitor started telling me I needed to stop pumping because the stress must be contributing to my mood. I told her that I didn't mind pumping at all. She talked over me to explain that being tied to a pump 8 times a day is a fast track to depression, and how could I enjoy my boys if all I was doing was pumping?
>
> I was so taken aback, I just nodded, said I'd think about it, and we moved on with the appointment. However, I was fuming all the way home. Pumping was not making me depressed. The biggest contributing factors to my depression were being a mum to a tricky 2-year-old and a 4-month-old who did nothing but scream (we later found out Oliver had CMPA and my eldest is autistic), while my husband worked 14-hour days and I had limited practical support and lived in the middle of nowhere. Expressing my milk was not a factor.

> So, when I was preparing for my IBCLC exam, and found the study that demonstrates breastfeeding isn't a cause of depression but not achieving our breastfeeding goals is. Well, that made so much sense to me and explained a lot about how the mums I was supporting felt as well (Brown, Rance, & Bennett, 2016).

There is a lot more to this than my experience. The science behind maternal mental health and lactation makes perfect sense. Breastfeeding parents have higher levels of oxytocin (it's triggered by the baby feeding), and oxytocin makes us feel all chilled out and dreamy. Oxytocin also suppresses the stress response, which lowers the risk of depression, anxiety, and other mental health conditions. Breastfeeding mums experience less stress compared to formula-feeding parents, and we all know that stress can negatively impact mood.

Breastfeeding Gives You Saggy Breasts

Genetics and pregnancy change your breasts, not breastfeeding. This is due to how the ligaments stretch in pregnancy. You don't tend to notice these changes while lactating because milk keeps them looking fuller and rounder, so it's not until lactation is over that people notice the change in their breast structure and end up thinking that breastfeeding was the cause.

If You Have Chickenpox, Stop Breastfeeding Until You're Well Again

Quick sidenote: In the UK, we don't vaccinate against chickenpox. I am aware that other countries do, however.

Chickenpox, or varicella-zoster virus is common in childhood in the UK. Most adults are immune to it, but not everyone is. Occasionally, a nursing parent will develop the virus and at this point, they will often be told to pump and dump their milk, or to express and bottle feed.

This is a bit pointless, as the virus is present and contagious for about 48 hours before the symptoms start to appear, meaning that the baby will have been exposed by the time Mum is itching. Official guidance is that it is better to carry on breastfeeding as normal. Babies past the newborn stage tend to cope well with chickenpox if they do get it, often getting fewer spots than their older siblings and just bobbing their way through the illness. Sadly, there is no evidence that chickenpox antibodies or other protective factors are present in Mum's milk.

If you spend 24 with a breastfed toddler and their parent, you will observe the child requesting milk, endlessly, and often, Mum saying, "not right now," or words to the same effect.

Stop Breastfeeding If You Have COVID-19 (Or Wear a Mask While Breastfeeding)

As with chickenpox, by the time you have symptoms of COVID-19, you're already contagious and your baby has already been exposed. While research on the impact of COVID on breastfeeding babies is still somewhat limited (I am writing this section in October 2021), when parents are sick, COVID antibodies are present in human milk, which protects infants. Most babies cope well if they do get COVID and experience a mild illness in most cases. Younger babies may suffer if Mum has to wear a mask during feeds because they can't see her face. Older babies either become distressed or distracted by masks, even trying to poke them or pull them off.

Pump and Dump If You Have a Stomach Virus or Food Poisoning

Your milk doesn't contain the virus or the bacteria making you sick; that's happening in your gut, not your bloodstream, where milk is made.

Continuing to breastfeed with a virus protects your baby against the illness, makes them less likely to get sick, and more likely to recover faster if they do catch the bug.

Your milk supply might decrease if you become dehydrated, but if you feel well enough to keep feeding responsively, your baby will get their needs met, just with more feeds than normal. Oral rehydration solutions are considered safe to take while breastfeeding and can help.

You Can't Breastfeed If You Have HIV

Breastfeeding with HIV is complicated, but I'll try to summarise. Studies show that when HIV+ mothers breastfeed exclusively, their risk of catching HIV from her are low if Mum is receiving antiretroviral therapy. However, if that baby is mixed-feeding, HIV transmission increases significantly. As such, UNICEF states that if formula is not acceptable, feasible, affordable, sustainable, and safe (as is often the case in areas where HIV transmission is high), exclusive breastfeeding is recommended.

The British HIV Association states that while HIV+ mothers in the UK should formula-feed from birth, they should also be supported to breastfeed if that is their wish. This is because the risk of transmission is low. Though, the mother would have to be taking antiretroviral therapy and submit to regular testing of her viral load. The British HIV Association also states that breastfeeding with HIV is not a safeguarding concern as long as she follows the previously listed requirements. If her tests begin to come back positive, she should stop breastfeeding, as this would present a safeguarding concern.

If Mum develops mastitis or damaged nipples, the risk of infection for her baby also increases, so *good* breastfeeding support is crucial.

There is lack of clarity regarding whether breastfeeding is safe once solids are introduced (remember, the risk is higher in babies not EBF). The UK recommends that mothers stop breastfeeding at 6 months. However, the WHO says that mothers should be encouraged to continue until 12 months, if they live someplace where formula is not safe, affordable, available, or an accessible option.

I've taken the information above from a combination of an LLL article called, "Breastfeeding and HIV," and in discussion with Pamela Morrison, IBCLC, an expert in this area. Her book on the topic of breastfeeding and HIV was published in 2022.

If You Have Cancer

No one wants to think about this, of course. However, cancer can happen at any time, and you may be more likely to discover breast cancer while breastfeeding because you are aware of your breasts and notice changes. Equally, it can be challenging to be diagnosed during lactation because it is more difficult to evaluate a breast full of milk. Let's address some myths about cancer and lactation.

- You Can Give Your Baby Cancer

Absolutely not. Cancer is not contagious, even breast cancer while breastfeeding. A mum with cancer does not increase her baby's risks of developing cancer.

- You Need to Stop Right Away

The diagnostic tests are safe for lactation, and some cancer treatments are also safe.

- You Must Stop for Radiotherapy

If your breast is receiving therapy, do not feed on that side. However, you can breastfeed from your other side as normal.

- Wean So You Can Focus on Recovery

Weaning is often highly distressing for mother and child, and if breastfeeding has been used as an overall parenting tool, then weaning will only make life harder for everyone involved.

The Drugs in Breastmilk Information Service can support you with your individual circumstances, as the above answers are generalised. Please seek extra help if you are diagnosed with cancer.

CHAPTER 9

Formula and Bottles

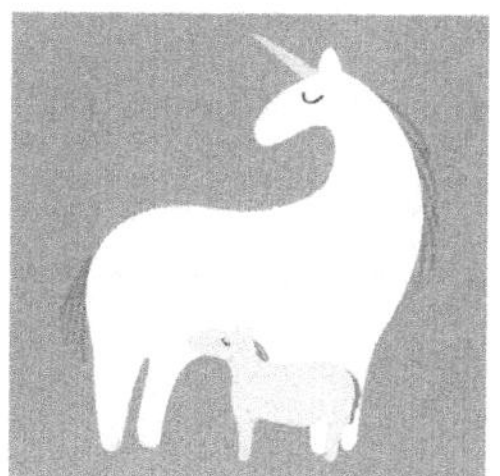

Formula Is Highly Specialised, Lab-Created Breastmilk

I wish it was because it would suggest that formula manufacturers cared more about babies' health than profits. Sadly, formula is essentially dried cows' milk (or soy) with added vitamins. It does a marvellous job of giving your baby the correct balance of nutrition, but it is nothing like breastmilk. Even when the company states that certain milks have special ingredients, or are softer on the stomach, no evidence backs up their claims. If they did, all formulas in the UK would be required to include these ingredients.

X Or Y Bottle Is the Closest to a Breast

Companies spend a lot of money telling us that their bottle is best, the closest to the breast, the easiest to switch to, and all sorts of other ridiculous claims ("anti-colic," I'm looking at you). Aside from their own customer feedback, which they share carefully ("80% of parents agree our bottle is..."), no evidence supports their claims.

When we consider different bottles, despite dozens of brands on the market, they fall into three categories: wide neck, narrow neck, and orthodontic. That's it. Everything else is a gimmick. Some professionals claim that a narrow-neck bottle is best. Some claim that the wide neck is best. These are all just opinions. There is no genuinely nonbiased evidence to support any of these claims. I suggest you use the bottle your baby will take, pace feeds, and use the slowest flowing teat that works for your baby.

Formula Will Make Your Baby Sleep More

Recent studies have shown your baby may sleep more if formula-fed, but you actually get less sleep (Dorheim et al., 2009; Kendall-Tackett et al., 2011). While more sleep for your baby might sound like a good thing, it is also a risk for SIDS (sudden infant death syndrome). Night-time waking is normal for babies, at least until the age of 2. A current theory of SIDS is that babies get into such a deep sleep that they cannot rouse, so waking protects them. Many infants wake at least two times per night well beyond their first birthday.

The real issue isn't infant sleep, but a lack of support for new parents. In an ideal world, someone would be around to take the burden off of new mums: to cook, clean, and hold the baby while Mum naps or rests. Unfortunately, we don't live in a culture that allows that for most families, so mums are more tired and babies' normal sleeping patterns are harder to deal with. They end up feeling like a problem that needs to be fixed.

Current evidence shows that breastfeeding mums get more sleep because they are not waking up in the same way as their formula-feeding counterparts. When a formula-fed baby wakes at night, a parent must get up, prepare formula, and then feed the baby. When a breastfed baby wakes, parents can often just pull their babies next to them, pop a boob out, and doze, all without leaving the bed if the baby is close by.

Formula Will Stop Your Baby from Crying Excessively

Formula can help if your baby is struggling with breastfeeding and needs more milk. However, in the meantime, parents need skilled breastfeeding support: feeding assessments, help expressing, and techniques to increase milk supply. We shouldn't just throw formula at a problem without getting to the root of it. Formula can even increase crying if your baby struggles to digest it, is allergic or sensitive to it, or if they overfeed.

Colic Formula Will Stop Colic

There is no evidence that colic formula makes any difference. Colic is a symptom that needs investigating, not masking with a thick milk. That's all anti-reflux/colic/comfort milks are—thickened infant milk. They can also make it harder for your baby to be sick, but won't necessarily resolve any underlying causes of their crying/fussing/pain.

Bottle-Feeding Will Cause Bottle Preference

There are downsides to bottles, for sure. In the West, they are something most parents are comfortable with because they are familiar and most people have used a bottle to feed a sibling, relative, or family friend's baby. We are beginning to think that bottles might not be so bad for nipple confusion, if they are used in a particular way. Paced bottle-feeding seems to reduce the chances of babies refusing the breast. This is probably because we keep the flow slow and pay close attention to hunger and satiety cues. We can further support the baby with suck training and finger-feeding exercises to strengthen sucking skills needed at the breast, maintaining a good milk supply, and working on underlying issues leading to bottle use.

Bottle feeding can cause breastfeeding difficulties, but they don't always and for babies needing a top up, it's not helpful to tell parents that bottles are adding to their problems, particularly if they aren't.

Formula Fixes Breastfeeding Problems

Formula often masks breastfeeding problems. If babies gain weight slowly, topping them up with formula won't tell us *why* they are struggling. Did they have a tongue-tie or suck dysfunction? Does Mum have a hormonal disorder? If formula is given to a fussy baby, we don't know if the behaviour is normal, the baby is unwell, Mum's milk is a bit fast, there's an allergy to consider, or there was anything else of concern.

Of course, formula may be needed (or wanted—choice is *really* important) but it should not be used as a metaphorical plaster for a gaping wound needing stitches.

The Formula Companies Want to Support Families

With their helplines, clubs, and freebies, formula companies are doing a good job of seeming like they want to help families. Unfortunately, this is about brand loyalty and selling a product, not genuine concern for your baby's health. Often, information they provide is unhelpful, inaccurate, or worded to place doubt in parents' minds when it comes to breastfeeding. You don't have to spend much time clicking around a formula-company website to find information that is:

- **Poorly Worded.** "Don't put too much pressure on yourself if you're unwell; try expressing so you can go back to breastfeeding when you're feeling better."
- **Over Complicated.** "Wash your hands before you start and have a glass of water close by. Get yourself comfortable by sitting down with your back straight and your lap flat. Pop a couple of cushions behind you to support your back. Use another cushion on your knees to help bring your baby closer to your breast, if needed."
- **Taken Out of Context.** "The nutritional choices you make enable your baby to get the vitamins and minerals they need to support their future health."

You might be thinking that as long as they're supporting formula-feeding families, that's the most important thing. You'd be right. I wonder how much money it costs them to write their breastfeeding articles and staff their carelines. They promote themselves as a source of infant-feeding support, including breastfeeding. They send emails about baby development, advertise follow-on milks, sponsor midwifery conferences, and send out toys and other gifts to pregnant women. If the goal was truly to support formula-feeding families, wouldn't it make more sense to spend that money on making formula healthier, helping more parents reach their infant-feeding goals, or ensuring that no one has to water down formula to make it last? After all, according to Baby Milk Action, 50% to 80% of the price is actually going on promotional campaigns.

I'll leave you with a few stories, which perfectly demonstrate the burden formula can leave people dealing with.

> *I was a teen mum on benefits with postnatal psychosis. I was getting £180 every two weeks to pay for everything. I couldn't afford formula. It was so bad, that as soon as my baby showed signs of CMPA, I begged my doctor to prescribe formula so I didn't have to pay for it and could spend the healthy start vouchers on food for me and my partner, just to survive. I am so upset looking back. I was so ill and broke. The system is so broken.* ◆ **Charlotte**

> *COVID has been particularly financially challenging to many already suffering and struggling South Africans.*
>
> *1. People who barely managed to afford formula simply had no money to even buy enough to stretch. With the simple result of concocting their own baby formulas, with any combination of cows' milk, milk powder, sugar, flour, rice, cereal, and canola oil. These recipes flooded the internet and even newspapers, and many moms found it a relief to not have to choose between feeding their family and feeding their baby anymore; they've "found the perfect middle ground."*
>
> *2. It's considered a "rich woman's life, being able to hold off solids for 4 to 6 months." They cannot afford storage for breastmilk, time for pumping, or other practicalities when returning to work (as early as 2*

weeks postpartum) any more than they can afford formula, and baby needs to survive on something.

3. When formula is running out, moms use pacifiers, water, tea, and cows' milk to stretch feeds until they are paid again.

4. South Africa, theoretically, has clinics where people can collect formula. These are government funded and they almost never get paid, and when they do, staff salaries, rent, electricity, etc. are priority over formula. They do advise moms to breastfeed but have zero training to support this. ◆ **Sune**

Please note that it is *not* recommended that you make your own formula. This can lead to significant problems for your baby.

Thankfully, we were lucky enough to have managed to find our way back to breastfeeding without stretching or watering formula down, but when my milk production was down, we actually had a shock and needed to go into our savings to afford basic needs for the baby (diapers, formula, clothing, etc). And we are two working professionals with decent salaries, but sadly, having one bread earner on SMP really pushes you to a limit here in the UK. ◆ **Teo**

CHAPTER 10

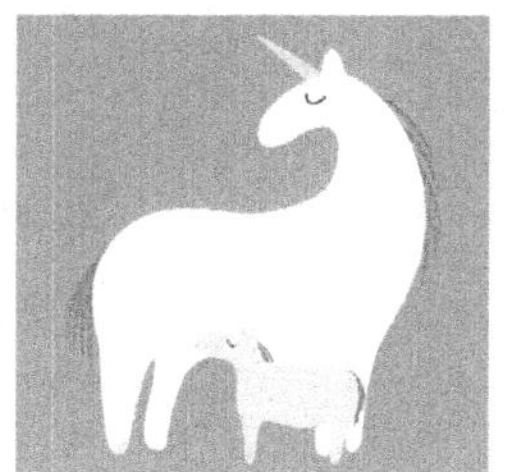

The Top Ten Weirdest Myths I've Heard

There isn't a huge amount to be said for most of the myths that follow here, but I wanted to include them to show the full scale of nonsense that exists about human milk and breastfeeding. At their best, they show a basic misunderstanding of how lactation works, and at their worst, they risk damaging a breastfeeding relationship.

Top Ten Weirdest Lactation Myths:

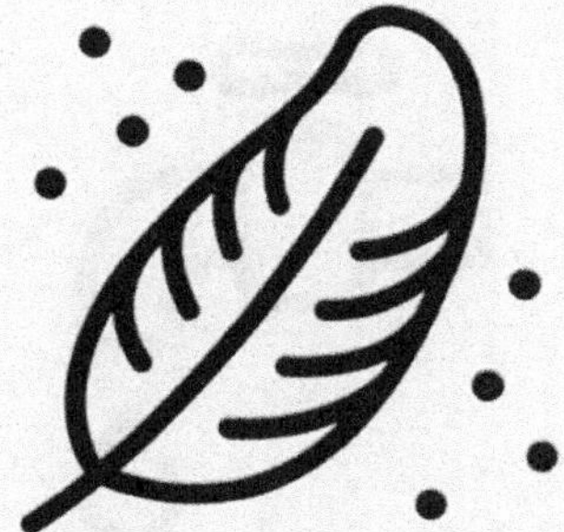

"Breastfeeding a boy will make him soft."

Top Ten Weirdest Lactation Myths:

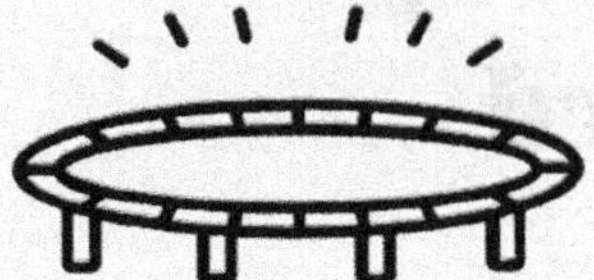

"Jumping on a trampoline will mix up your milk."

Top Ten Weirdest Lactation Myths:

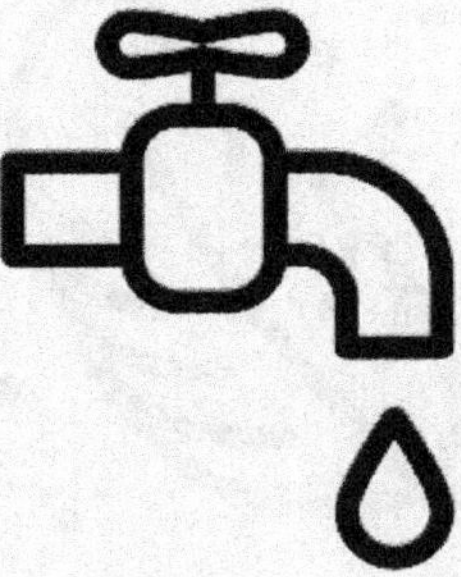

"Throw out foremilk, it's just water ."

Top Ten Weirdest Lactation Myths:

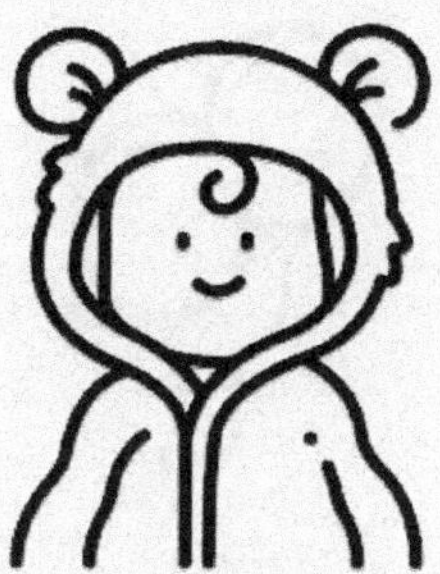

"Breastfeeding beyond (Arbitrary age) is a safeguarding concern ."

Top Ten Weirdest Lactation Myths:

"Your breastfed girl will be a lesbian."

Top Ten Weirdest Lactation Myths:

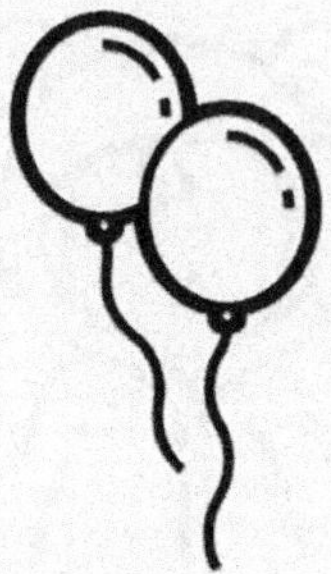

"If your baby falls asleep on the breast they will blow air back into the ducts and give you mastitis."

Top Ten Weirdest Lactation Myths:

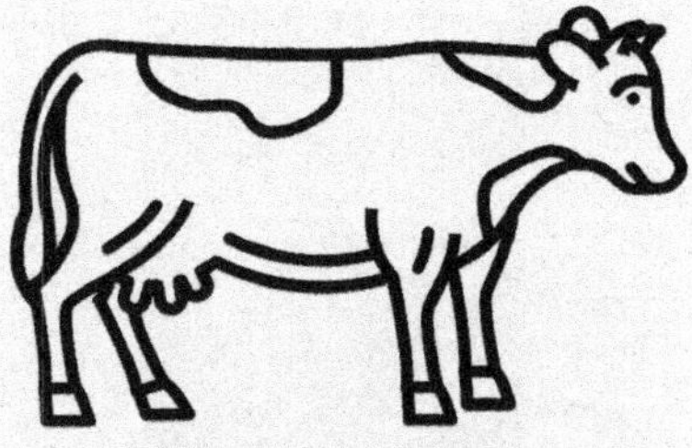

"Human milk is weird and gross - Giving them milk for a baby cow is ok though."

Top Ten Weirdest Lactation Myths:

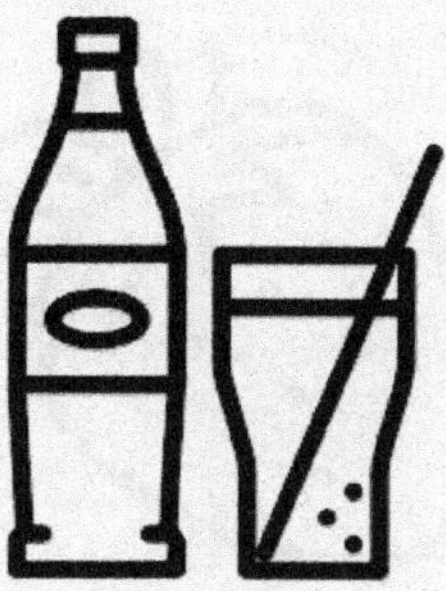

"Soda bubbles can get into your milk and make baby gassy."

Top Ten Weirdest Lactation Myths:

"Sunbathing will make your milk go sour."

Top Ten Weirdest Lactation Myths:

"If you eat strawberries the seeds will get into your milk."

CHAPTER 11

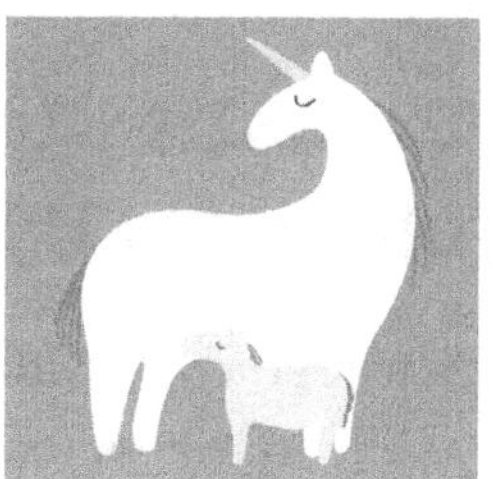

Truths That Sound Like Myths

I think this is a good place to focus on some more of the amazing things breastmilk can do and provide, rather than the nonsense people misunderstand or make up about it. These are some of my personal favourite facts that tend to make people look at me a bit sideways and say, "Really?"

Breastfeeding Parents Are Less Tired Than Their Formula-Feeding Friends

A 2007 study found that if you're breastfeeding, both you and your partner get more sleep than your peers who are formula feeding. They report an average of an extra 45 minutes sleep each night for breastfeeding parents, which doesn't sound like a big deal, but the study goes on to explain that just 30 minutes of extra awake time can have a negative impact on how you feel and function (Doan et al., 2007). Two more recent studies, with larger samples, also found that exclusively breastfeeding mothers got more sleep, were less fatigued, and were less likely to get depressed than their formula- and mixed-feeding peers (Dorheim et al., 2009; Kendall-Tackett et al., 2011). Exclusively breastfed babies wake more often, but mothers go back to sleep more quickly. If you are breastfeeding, you don't typically need to get out of bed to feed; you can just sit up, lift your baby from their cot, and you might even feed lying down, meaning that you continue to doze during feeds.

Breastmilk Can Help Clear Up Eye Infections

A 2021 study found that using breastmilk in babies' gunky eyes was just as effective as standard eye drops in clearing up the infection (Sugimura et al., 2021).

Every Drop Counts

If you've read my other books, or seen much of my social media, you will know that topic is important to me. While it's true that the more human milk given, the better the outcomes, there are good reasons to give your baby *any* amount of breastmilk. The longer you do so, the better it is. A teaspoon has 3 million germ-killing cells in it—in just 5ml of milk! If you cannot produce a full supply, or your baby doesn't latch, you could give small amounts of your milk in a syringe, like medicine. It's little shots of antibodies a few times a day.

If your baby is happy to latch, despite a low supply/no supply, it's helps them too. Sucking helps to calm babies, as does being skin-to-skin (cheek-to-breast counts) with you. They will be taking small amounts of milk, which is made up from your own immune system, therefore protective against any viruses you or your baby have encountered.

Your Breasts Change Temperature, Depending on Your Baby's Needs

This fact sounds so incredible that people assume it's a myth. If you have twins, one on each breast, your breasts will independently adjust their temperature, depending on what each baby needs. If one baby is chilly, one breast will warm up for them, and if the other is warm, that breast will cool down.

You Can Restart a Milk Supply After Years of Not Feeding

This is another topic close to my heart. Relactation, the work of rebuilding a milk supply after a gap but without a new pregnancy, is absolutely possible, even years later. Breast stimulation with a baby or a pump, along with herbs and/or prescription medication can make relactation a possibility. I did it myself, although after weeks, not months. I have also supported countless others. Some parents breastfed an adopted baby several years after breastfeeding their birth children. Results are mixed, and a full supply might not always be possible, but most parents can produce some milk. Often a significant amount. In one case study, a grandmother relactated to feed her grandson after his mum died of malaria (Patnaik, 1999).

You Can Lactate and Never Be Pregnant

Just like relactation is possible, induced lactation is as well. It typically involves prescription medications, but not always. Results can vary from just a few drops to a full supply. Yes, you can lactate and never be pregnant.

You Can Exclusively Breastfeed Triplets

It's not easy, but it has been done many times. At least three studies discuss this topic. A Canadian study looked at nine mothers with triplets. Five of them managed to exclusively (or nearly exclusively) breastfeed for between 2 and 7 months (Leonard, 2000). Mead et al. (1992) describe a case where quadruplets were exclusively breastfed (they fed up to 13 times a day).

Breastmilk Significantly Improves the Outcomes for Preemies

If you have a premature baby, you will be actively encouraged to provide them with your milk while they are in the NICU, at least until they reach their due date. There are many reasons why your milk, or donor milk, is especially important for preemies. All of them significantly improve the babies' outcomes.

For example, there is an illness called necrotising enterocolitis (NEC), which premature infants are particularly at risk of developing. NEC is a condition where the bowel becomes inflamed, and this leads to damage and eventually, death of the tissue. Feeding premature babies only human milk reduces the chances of NEC by 6 to10 times. In the absence of Mum's own milk, donor milk has similar outcomes.

Milk from a parent feeding a preemie is higher in sodium, chloride, and nitrogen than full-term milk, and has a higher ratio of immunological factors. All these things are especially important for preemies.

Human milk feeding can also help prepare babies for oral feeding by building enteral tolerance, and it is often used in mouth care (where babies mouths are moistened), which helps them develop positive associations with the taste of human milk.

When You Breastfeed, You Share Your Immune System with Your Baby

Your milk has white blood cells in it, and white blood cells are a key part of your immune system. One million white blood cells are present in each drop of breastmilk (Zhou et al., 2000). These white blood cells survive the passage into the baby's gut and then move to other places where needed, such as the liver. Leukocytes (a type of white blood cell) fight unwanted or foreign cells present in the baby's body and support babies' developing immune system. As an interesting side note, the human immune system doesn't work on its own until middle childhood. This is why some think that children are designed to breastfeed until the milk teeth fall out, around 6 years of age (Simon et al., 2015).

CHAPTER 12

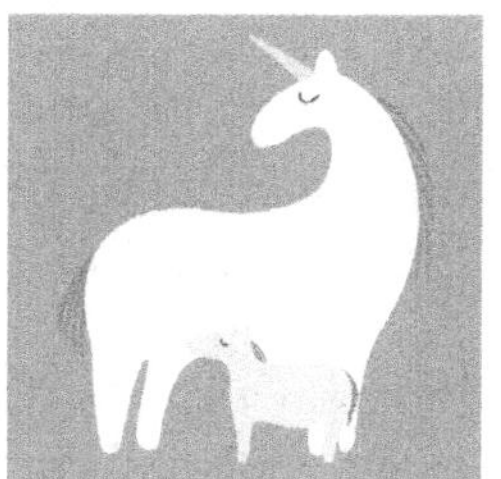

Myths around Underrepresented Parents

Transgender

Terms Like Chestfeeding Are Eliminating Women-Centred Language

In recent years, inclusive language around lactation has increased. According to the trans and nonbinary communities, language regarding body anatomy causes significant feelings of distress, trauma, or shame. Adding in more neutral terms, such as chestfeeding, lactation, human milk feeding, or body feeding alongside the more traditional breastfeeding can make a huge difference to parents who are dealing with difficult feelings daily.

Some worry that inclusive language will replace gendered terms like mother or woman, and therefore, using nonbinary words is not appropriate. In October 2021, I went to five well-known breastfeeding-focused social media pages, including well-established charities. I looked at the last five posts on each page and counted how many of those posts mentioned "mother" or "breastfeeding," and how many used a gender-neutral term such as "chestfeeding," "parent," or "lactation" instead.

Out of over 25 posts, 22 of them expressly mentioned mother, breastmilk, or breastfeeding. Only three used gender-neutral terms, and two of those did this as well as the women-centred language above. That leaves us with one single post out of 25 across five different charities and organisations that was deliberately nonbinary. I suggest that fears around women being erased from lactation are somewhat overstated.

Some say that the term "breastfeeding" is the best way to describe feeding a baby with your body, because everyone has breast tissue, regardless of gender. However, this dismisses the fact that many trans and nonbinary people find discussion of breasts distressing. You could argue the other way: we all have breast tissue on our chests.

To be serious, respecting the language individuals want to use shouldn't be controversial or difficult. Once we overcome the myth that women are being removed from lactation, we can all do this a lot more clearly.

Finally, we assume gender-neutral language only serves the trans or nonbinary community, but there is a huge place for it in terms of sexual abuse survivors as well. I don't think anyone would argue against a child sexual abuse survivor requesting that a neutral term such as "chest" or "lactation" is used within their care if it helps to avoid the trigger of gendered language.

The Trans Community Hate Their Bodies So Why Would They Want to Lactate?

Body dysphoria is incredibly complex, but it isn't the same as hating your body. As a ciswoman with a history of body dysphoria, I loved breastfeeding because it gave my body a function that had nothing to do with its appearance. Many trans folk report the same. You can be uncomfortable in your body but still want to use it to help grow your baby. It is certainly not a given that a transperson hates their body. Many don't. Here are some moving words from Tez (they/them) about this topic:

> I knew when they arrived, these soft round things, that while they were lovely, they were not designed to be on my body. When I asked the doctor to remove them in my early teens, he told me I would need them to feed my babies one day and he was right. Feeding my babies with milk from my breasts was both the hardest and most rewarding thing I ever did. Feeding my babies from my body

became an act of resistance, a way to break generational patterns. As for my littles, I knew they needed it.

I marvelled at the way fluid from my body could grow humans, how using them as a parenting tool soothed us all. I fed though pregnancy and then nourished two children until they were both over 4. I dealt with the dysphoria by learning about how and why lactation happened. It became my specialism in my work.

The milk from my body met the kids' needs for allergy-safe milk; it met their neurodivergent needs. They offered comfort and safety over a time in their life that they had little. It came at a cost for me, with many technical issues and severe aversion. But the breasts, they did the thing they needed to do. I saw them as on loan and they worked hard for us.

Now that my children are weaned, the dysphoria has shifted again. My mammaries did their job and I plan to yeet them, with love, into oblivion when it is practically possible. My children got a better parent for the fact I learn to live with the dysphoria. I do not hate them; I love them on others; they just don't belong on me.

The Testosterone Transmen Take Is Dangerous to Their Baby

Trans folk stop taking their testosterone when they become pregnant, or if they are planning to carry and birth a baby. We see far less outrage when ciswomen are taking the contraceptive pill and fall pregnant. Testosterone doesn't make a transman infertile either, which is important to note, as some people will say pregnancy and lactation is not appropriate for a transman, as they "should" be infertile.

You Can't Lactate If You're a Man

Firstly, at least one cisman, using the medication and a pumping schedule, was able to induce lactation. Secondly, if you were born into a body that grew breasts and milk-making tissue, you can lactate if you haven't had top surgery. Thirdly, if you don't have any mammary gland tissue (either because you had it removed or never had any), you could use a supplementing nursing system to feed your baby at your chest, even if the milk passing through the tube is donor milk or formula. Feeding your baby with your body is a lot more than milk production. Your baby will feel safe, warm, and relaxed while nursing with you, and that is one of the most incredible things we can give our babies.

The Milk Transwomen Make Is Harmful to Their Infant, Due to the Drugs Used to Induce Lactation

The drugs in question (the contraceptive pill and domperidone) are widely used in ciswomen who are breastfeeding and there are no risks associated for their babies. Why would a transwoman be any different?

You Can't Feed with Your Body If You've Had Top Surgery

You can use a feeding tube and maybe a nipple shield to allow your baby to nurse at your chest, even if you don't have any glandular tissue. However, many people still have some glandular tissue after top surgery. It's similar to the same way a ciswoman can lactate after having breast surgery. A transman may still be able to lactate.

You Can't Breastfeed a Baby You Didn't Birth

Yes, you can. Whether you are adopting or want to co-breastfeed with the birth parent, if you have working breast tissue, you can probably lactate, even without pregnancy. Induced lactation can be a tricky journey, but it has been done many times.

In addition, no evidence suggests that using your body to feed a baby you haven't birthed is problematic for you or your little one. People have helped to feed other mothers' babies since the dawn of humankind, and it's normal in many cultures.

Autism Spectrum Disorders and Sensory Processing Disorders

Autism spectrum disorders make some aspects of day-to-day life more challenging. Women are typically underdiagnosed and present differently than men. This means that a lot of mothers don't know that they are on the spectrum, or maybe have a new diagnosis, after spending much of their childhood and adolescence feeling, somehow, wrong. Symptoms of autism spectrum disorders include difficulties with communication, a need for structure and routine, and a strong sense of right and wrong.

Additionally, Sensory Processing Disorder (SPD) and Pathological Demand Avoidance (PDA) often go hand in hand with autism spectrum disorders. As a result, some professionals assume that an autistic parent either won't breastfeed because of the demand, or will breastfeed, even if it's detrimental to their own health, because it is what you are "supposed" to do.

I asked the #actuallyautistic community about this and met with a similar range of views. The West tries to put people into boxes according to diagnoses, which is incredibly unhelpful. Some people said that breastfeeding was challenging due to their autism. At the top of the list was sensory overload. However, many said that they enjoyed breastfeeding, especially once the extreme unpredictability of the newborn days eased up.

A few people said that they started breastfeeding so they could stick to the "rules," and breastfed longer than they wanted through a sense of guilt. When I dug a little deeper, these feelings seemed to reflect the available support, not the experience of breastfeeding per se. In a few cases, parents assumed that they had to carry on because their supporters were breastfeeding older children and only talked about ways to continue through challenges. One mum told me:

> If someone had said that I could stop, I would have. I was afraid that if I didn't carry on, I would be judged as a bad parent, and that's something I was already dealing with as an autistic mother.

I also learned that anxiety is high in parents with autism, but they are also motivated to make breastfeeding work. If breastfeeding doesn't work, there is more feelings of failure, guilt, and shame. Parents with autism usually read a lot about breastfeeding, which makes it more frustrating and upsetting when it doesn't work. Parents said that compassionate, reliable, honest, and clear breastfeeding support is essential for dealing with challenges and any difficult feelings they experience.

A significant number of people said that their sensory processing differences made breastfeeding harder, but not enough to stop breastfeeding.

In summary, breastfeeding with autism spectrum disorders is not black and white. Sweeping statements about whether they will breastfeed are unhelpful and inaccurate, particularly without context. As there is little research, the experience of breastfeeding as a person with autism becomes more important than usual.

Parents with Sensory Processing Disorders Should Just Try Distraction Techniques

Sensory Processing Disorder (SPD), or any sensory processing differences, manifest as either a need for extra stimulation or an over sensitivity to stimulation. Some people can experience both. For example, someone with SPD may find noise unbearable, but may need the deep pressure of a weighted blanket.

The physical sensations of breastfeeding can feel overwhelming. Anyone who has experienced aversion will know the nails-on-chalkboard feeling that a shallow latch or endless feed can bring.

If you recognise the challenges with sensory processing, does distraction help? It can, but there is more to consider. Sensory overload isn't just about breastfeeding; everything becomes heightened when your senses are on alert. Noises become more jarring, light becomes brighter, and a cluttered room screams at you.

Many parents with SPD find that headphones, low lights, and a weighted blanket help more than distraction techniques and mindfulness. Damping down the alert system can help to calm Mum so that feeding is less overpowering.

Some parents report being well hydrated and not hungry before feeds can help, as can limiting conflicting background noise. Being physically relaxed is worth exploring, so is listening to meditation. Using hypnosis might also be helpful. Personally, I found mindfulness made my symptoms worse, but focusing on my breathing and a guided meditation story was helpful.

Attention-Deficit/Hyperactivity Disorder (ADHD)

ADHD Medication Is Not Safe for Breastfeeding

As is often the case with medication and breastfeeding, the drugs prescribed for attention-deficit/ hyperactivity disorder (ADHD) have not been well studied in regard to lactation. The Drugs in Breastmilk Information Service in the UK explains that for methylphenidate (Concerta/ Ritalin), atomexatine, and lisdexamphatime (Vyvanse), small amounts pass through breastmilk, but "may not affect the infant adversely." They note the a lack of research and advise that parents watch the baby for agitation, poor feeding, and poor sleep when taking ADHD medication.

> *I have ADHD and was told I had to wean before starting medication. I did research and talked to Wendy at the Drugs in Breastfeeding Service, and found I didn't.* ◆ **Bethan**

On the other hand, proving it's never straightforward:

> *The BFN (Breastfeeding Network sent me info on all the studies that have been done, and they are so limited. The number of participants is tiny, and none of the studies tracked the child's development past 12 months. My psychiatrist was very reluctant due to how limited the research was, and after checking it out myself, at the time, I agreed, as there were some effects noted in the studies. I guess it's a case of personal choice based on limited data until any further research is done (if it ever is).* ◆ **Jenn**

I like Jenn's final thought about personal choice being based on limited data. Also consider to extent to which ADHD is affecting your life. Simply refusing breastfeeding mothers' medication is problematic. I'd love it if we could, oh, I don't know, be trusted to review the available information and come up with our own conclusions.

Someone With ADHD Will Hate Breastfeeding Because They Have to Sit Still for a Long Time

Attention-deficit/hyperactivity disorder is another condition woefully underdiagnosed in girls and women. When we think of ADHD, we imagine "naughty" schoolboys rampaging through a classroom, but we don't think of girls hair-twiddling, wandering around the water fountain, forgetting homework, losing a PE kit, and being talkative. Girls learn to mask our symptoms very well, very early on.

I have ADHD and I loved breastfeeding. My ADHD primarily manifests as inattentiveness and daydreaming! Breastfeeding meant I didn't have to think about the million things I needed to do. All I needed to do was respond when my baby needed me. Boob, clean nappy, and sleep. It was so simple (once I got to grips with it). Caring for a baby full time pushed out a lot of noise in my head about work, cleaning, groceries, etc. For me, lactation became what's known in the ADHD world as a hyperfocus (where we focus all of our energy on one particular thing; researching, reading, total emersion). This is why, 8 years later, I am writing my third book on the topic. Of course, I was hugely privileged to have a partner who took on a lot of the extra stuff. Not everyone has that, and not everyone with ADHD has my experience of breastfeeding.

When I spoke with people in the ADHD community about whether it was true that they wouldn't breastfeed because they needed to move around, they expressed their frustration with society's assumptions about us. A few mums said this rang somewhat true for them, but not to the point where they didn't want to breastfeed anymore. They talked about using their phones or a TV show as distractions, or learning to breastfeed while walking around, often with the aid of a sling. I spoke with lots of parents in generic social media groups to avoid only getting people who loved breastfeeding. They told me that, as in my case, breastfeeding became an obsession or hyperfocus. Many ADHDers trained as peer supporters, breastfeeding counsellors, and IBCLCs. In fact, it was hard to find people with ADHD who said that it made breastfeeding harder for them.

Women Who Have Been Abused Don't Want to Breastfeed

Before I was an IBCLC, I worked alongside professionals who had a lot of contact with new parents. I vividly remember that one member of the team said that we shouldn't ask a particular mother about breastfeeding because of her history of abuse. They didn't want to risk upsetting her. I also see this sentiment on social media and it's been brought up when I've trained volunteers. As with many things, it's a well-meaning approach, but does it reflect what parents need or want?

One large study found earlier breastfeeding cessation when women experienced abuse as children or adults (Sorbo et al., 2015). However, other studies have found similar rates of breastfeeding, and even exclusive breastfeeding for abuse survivors (Coles et al., 2016; Kendall-Tackett et al., 2013).

A qualitative study interviewed 6 childhood sexual abuse survivors about their breastfeeding experiences. All wanted to breastfeed, but all experienced challenges related to shame, dissociation, and touch. However, 2 women described breastfeeding as healing. This study concludes that compassionate care from professionals could improve breastfeeding outcomes for abuse survivors (Wood & van Esterik, 2010).

It felt important to include real life stories in this section. When I reached out on social media, I was blown away by the number of responses. I have included as many as I can below, but please take this as a *trigger warning* for discussion of abuse in many forms. Skip these stories if you need to protect your own mental wellness. I would also like to thank every single person who came forward to discuss this difficult and important topic with me.

Anonymous

I was sexually abused as a child, emotionally abused, and neglected by my mum (wasn't intentional; she, unfortunately, was also abused as a child and didn't know how to parent). I went on to have a relationship, which was violent. I ended the relationship after he caused me to miscarry.

At 21, I had my first child (a girl) with my now-husband. While pregnant, I was adamant I was going to breastfeed. I was going to be everything my mum couldn't be. After birth, I had no support from friends, family, midwives, etc. I put so much pressure on myself to be perfect that I stopped eating and sleeping. I stayed awake all night to clean, etc. At 3 days old, my baby had lost 10% of her birthweight, so the midwife told me I had to top her up with formula or else she would have to go into hospital. I felt like I had failed her. I topped up. However, very quickly, I found that she wasn't latching on to my breast, so I ended up formula-feeding her. I was later told I had PND, which more than likely was caused by the pressure I put on myself to be everything my mum couldn't be. I had a strong bond with my baby but couldn't let anyone else near her. I was the only one allowed to bath her, I would watch my husband change her nappy, etc.

My second child, a boy, was born 3 years later. It was a difficult pregnancy; I bled throughout. When he was born, he was so tiny, I refused to try to breastfeed him, as I was terrified of messing up again. I, again, put an insane amount of pressure on myself after finding out that my mum had told people that I would never cope with another child. He was an easy baby, but I felt something wasn't right with him. We later found out that he has a very rare genetic disorder. I still feel guilt for not trying to breastfeed him.

When I had my third child, another boy, I didn't entertain the idea of breastfeeding; the thought made me physically sick, not because of the sexual abuse, but because I was terrified of failing.

My fourth and final child, a girl, was born 4 years ago. She was formula-fed until a week old. We noticed she was very sickly. In fact, she projectile vomited an entire feed. She has a cows' milk protein allergy. At 6 days old, she was screaming in pain; I was crying with her. Nothing would calm her down. I don't know why, but I put her to my breast. She latched on, and we laid on the bed like that for ages. It was the calmest she had been. I decided, from then on, to breastfeed. It was hard; I took fenugreek; if I wasn't pumping, I was trying to latch her on the breast. I was exhausted, but I knew I had to do it. She was much calmer, and I felt incredible. I didn't get PND with her (I did with the other three). She is 4 now, and still breastfeeds. I wish I had had support with my other three children, as breastfeeding has helped to heal me. I finally feel like a mum and like I haven't messed something up.

Nicola

I wanted to breastfeed primarily for bonding with my baby. I understand the potential benefits for both mum and baby, but I was more focussed on promoting mental health in my baby.

Once I started breastfeeding, my reason for wanting to continue was more for the immune health benefits because I had my baby during the COVID-19 pandemic (June 2020).

I don't think my decision to breastfeed was consciously influenced by the abuse I experienced. But on reflection, I was aware of the theory of trauma being passed to future generations and wanting to break the cycle (I still strongly feel this way).

I had to stop sooner than planned. I did not get the support from the NHS because of COVID restrictions but I was fortunate enough to be able to afford an IBCLC. The IBCLC did a lot of work with me but the main thing I remember was her making me feel validated. At a time when I was struggling mentally, this was everything. She also followed up months after I had stopped paying for her service. With her support, I was able to get an ENT referral to another NHS Trust out of area and my babe had three lots of attempts at releasing her 'thick, tethering, anterior tongue-tie,' but unfortunately it was not resolved. I did mix feed, which was okay until my baby eventually lost interest in the effort of breastfeeding, which I expected to happen.

I didn't find it healing. The sensation of her at my breast actually made me angry and I had to squeeze something and distract myself, which took away all the bonding benefits I hoped for. Then, I felt guilty for feeling angry. Feelings were mixed between sadness, relief, and failure when breastfeeding ceased. I actually hand expressed right until I could only get one drop out into the teat of her bottle because I thought of the immune benefits of that one drop. Eventually, that became triggering and frustrating too, but it was easier to come to terms with stopping that.

This was an awful experience overall for me and I still have sensitivity in my nipples a year after stopping breastfeeding where, if something rubs against them, I get the same anger feeling for a second.

But, I am now proud of the start I gave my daughter, and I am proud of her for really trying to feed from me, despite her tongue-tie. She remains under SALT (Speech and Language Therapy) and may still need surgery when she is around 5 so maybe our experience is a little different, but I do wonder if any other survivors can relate to my feelings.

I made sure I took lots of photos at the time so I could look back with rose-tinted glasses and I love our bf selfies! I am very close with my little girl now. We have a lovely bond. Who knows? Maybe I didn't feel at the time but maybe the fight together did help us bond.

Emma

I was a victim of emotional abuse when I had my first daughter. I chose to breastfeed because I knew the health benefits behind this. I also loved the science behind it all and how it helped my relationship with her, and it had healing qualities and all that fun stuff. I actually breastfed my daughter until she was almost 3, and I actually did this, I think, looking back so that my ex-partner couldn't take her alone, as she needed me for feeds as her comfort. Her emotional needs became my number one priority in making sure she never suffered or felt I wasn't meeting her needs, and I did this through breastfeeding. However, I did live in fear that this would be taken from her with threats of court and solicitors all the time. I was told that because she was on solids, "she didn't need to breastfeed from me," so therefore, the courts could have granted overnight visits, etc., or even ordered me to stop if they felt it was interfering with their relationship. This was terrifying for me, as I felt it was the only way I was keeping my daughter protected and was able to meet her needs. Luckily, nothing like this happened and it was all just threats. However, it was a really horrific time in my life and it shocked me to the core that the courts can order such a thing without even looking at a situation because they didn't have time to look into every case and look into the needs of every specific child.

Amy

What was interesting, looking back, is that because my ex had a very detached and authoritarian parenting style, it made me lean massively away towards a very strongly attachment-based parenting style, almost too much. With my later two children that I had in a more supportive and healthy relationship, although I still believe broadly in AP, I was much more relaxed about things like mixed-feeding, not aggressively protecting my cosleeping status, sometimes prioritising myself over the baby, leaving them with other people, etc. With my first, it's like I felt I had to defend myself and my parenting all the time, so I became very rigid about how I did things according to a style rather than just what worked in the moment. I felt this was necessary in order to insulate my child from his father's parenting, which I felt was potentially damaging. I did feel that breastfeeding, cosleeping, using slings, gentle parenting, etc. was healing for my child—not as such for me. It wasn't bad for me, but it wasn't a way that I healed from that relationship. Although being confident in my parenting has helped me heal, in general, from some of the effects of that time.

Rebecca

> I saw your post about abuse and thought I might mention CPTSD (Complex Posttraumatic Stress Disorder), which a lot of people are suffering due to many different reasons—a lot of people can suffer with CPTSD and not necessarily realise due to how they were parented—emotional/mental abuse/neglect, etc.
>
> Not just strictly physical (though, I know you didn't specify that).
>
> I have managed to breastfeed for nearly 6 years consecutively, one child till 3.5 years old and the other is 2 years old, nearly 3. I suffer with really bad aversion and I suspect I feel touched out more quickly than others potentially do.
>
> I find reading a book on my phone or something is a good distraction for when aversion is strong.
>
> Also, I think dissociation probably plays a part in feeling connected to others and contributes to PND, etc., which I think can potentially affect the feeling of being able to connect or share my body, etc.

You Can't Breastfeed If You Have a Physical Disability

My first reaction to this is "why on Earth not?" The list of concerns that I've heard includes:

- It's too much for the parent to manage
- They don't have enough physical support around
- They aren't strong enough/mobile enough

As is usually the case, these ideas are typically well-intentioned but are rarely formed through talking to the people involved.

Mums with disabilities have two main concerns with regard to breastfeeding: positioning and attachment worries, and concerns about medications. Both can be overcome with good information and support the same way that we would support *anyone* with these issues. A less-common breastfeeding position might be needed, so that's why I recommend seeing a breastfeeding supporter. They can help you find the best position for you and your baby.

Breastfeeding also offers advantages when you have a disability. Here's what some families have told me:

- It's not as fiddly as preparing bottles when I have poor fine motor skills.
- It's easier at night.
- I don't have to carry the extra weight of bottles with me when I go out.
- I'm reducing my baby's chances of becoming unwell, which would be harder for me to deal with.
- I don't need to measure MLs and scoops with my poor eyesight.
- I never know how long my appointments will be, but I don't have to worry about not taking enough formula.
- I don't have a lot of control over many aspects of my life, but people have to let me feed my baby if I'm using my breasts to do so.

CHAPTER 13

Real Quotes from Real Parents

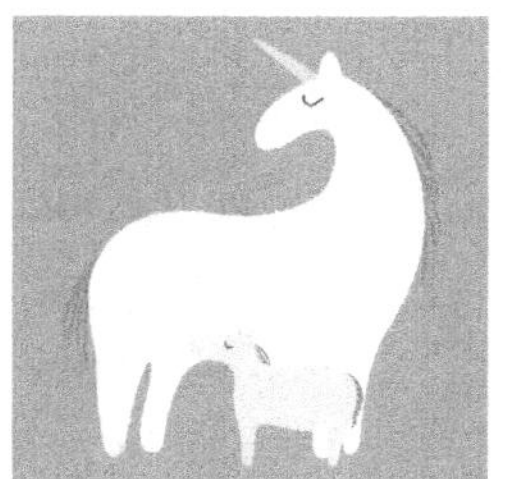

When I asked my Facebook community to tell me the myths they have encountered, I initially just wanted to use their quotes throughout the book but there are so many, covering so many random areas, that I decided to collate them here, instead. I'd say enjoy, but well, you'll see. A friend was told this:

> *I've never heard of anyone successfully breastfeeding a baby girl but maybe if the baby was a lesbian, that would work!"* ◆ **Ebony**

The global statistics for exclusive breastfeeding strongly suggest that plenty of (straight) baby girls are breastfed.

Exclusive breastfeeding (percent of children) under six months - UNICEF

- Croatia: 98%
- Rwanda: 86%
- Chile: 84%
- Zambia: 72%
- Nepal: 65%
- India: 54%
- Brazil: 41%

In addition, a 1993 study noted that most lesbians were not even aware of same-sex attraction until the age of 10. And they didn't identify as gay until they were around age 16, on average (Herdt & Boxer, 1993).

I received a letter, following a consult with an ENT surgeon, suggesting that the cause of all my nipple damage was not my twin boy's posterior tongue-tie but, perhaps, the simple fact that I was feeding twins. ◆ **Emma**

Once again here, we need to remember that good positioning and attachment should not cause pain, no matter how many babies you are feeding, because the nipple should be resting against the soft palate, and the equally soft tongue. Pain is typically caused by a nipple being pinched in a hard palate further forward in the mouth, and/or the tongue not covering the baby's lower gum. These issues are either caused by poor positioning and attachment, or are an underlying issue for your baby, such as tongue-tie.

A doctor told me exclusively pumping was pointless and at 9 months old, I was wasting my time. It was only important because I was "hormonal." ◆ **Amber**

It seems that no one has collected data on just how many parents exclusively express, but my own practice tells me it isn't an insignificant number. I know of many mums who pumped for 6, 12, 18 months, or even 2 years. Breastmilk from a pump is still a living organism, adapted to the environment the mother is in (and likely the environment her baby is in as well). This means that there are antibodies in that milk, as well as a near complete source of nutrition for a 9-month-old. As for the "you're just hormonal" stance, there are few statements so dismissive, undermining, and misogynist.

Some random woman I was buying carpets from in 2004 when pregnant with my eldest:

"You need to toughen up your nipples with a scourer."

I didn't, I was not that stupid. ◆ **Elly**

Thankfully, as Elly alludes to in her last sentence here, the practice of rubbing nipples (particularly with a scrub pad) to toughen them up is outdated. It doesn't help, but will make your nipples sore.

> *Paediatric lead at my local hospital told me allergens don't pass through breastmilk and my baby's poor weight gain was because I had hypoplasia. He threatened to report me to social services for intentionally starving my child if I didn't give cows' milk formula or wean at 5 months. Went on to prove 18 allergies, including cows' milk, and she thrived from that point on.* ◆ **Hayley**

> *It can't be CMPA because allergens can't travel through breastmilk. So, I ignored the GP, cut dairy from my diet and, lo and behold, my son stopped screaming every night, could be laid down on his back, stopped pooing mucous 12 times a day.* ◆ **Johanna**

The Drugs in Breastmilk Information Service's factsheet on Cow's Milk Protein Allergy says that 0.5% of breastfed babies have CMPA. This is because, despite Hayley's paediatrician and Johanna's GP claiming otherwise, allergens can and do pass from mum's diet into breastmilk. The percent of breastfed babies with CMPA is smaller than it is for formula-fed babies (up to 7.5% of these little ones have CMPA). Allergens are diluted by Mum before they are passed along, but it is a real issue that many dyads have to deal with.

> *I was told that I had to stop breastfeeding my son, as he was due for major surgery. I'd had a very traumatic BF experience anyway, as he would only direct feed at night, and I pumped like Daisy the cow all day, yet often, I would end up throwing it out. So, in the weeks leading up to the op, I stopped, only to have the nurses in HDU post-op telling me I could have continued with support from them. This made me sad.* ◆ **Sara**

Breastmilk is usually classed as a clear fluid, meaning most hospital settings will allow your baby to be breastfed up to 2 hours before any major surgery. There is no need to reduce or limit breastmilk ahead of surgery.

> *I was told that the reason for my first baby's awful reflux was because she "was greedy" by my health visitor and to restrict feeds. She had many other symptoms of a tongue-tie, which at the time, I was unfamiliar with. Its only since having my second who had a bad tongue-tie that I have been able to understand the most likely cause of why she was so unhappy that first year. I wish I had seen a lactation consultant*

with her, as things could've been so different for us instead of being fobbed off constantly and made to feel like a neurotic mother. ◆ **Kirsty**

We discuss this in more detail in the tongue-tie sections, but babies are not greedy. They are good at knowing when they are full or hungry, because they haven't learned to override their satiety cues from their stomachs yet, unlike many adults!

I can't prescribe you anything (for an injured wrist) because you're breastfeeding, and at 9 months, he's too old for it anyway, so come back when he's weaned. ◆ **Lucy**

Review the section on medication for more on this. Most pain medications are fine to take while breastfeeding, and you can talk to the Drugs in Breastmilk Information Service for more information if you're not sure.

I was told my baby would need formula top ups because she was premature. I successfully breastfed her (and still am at 2.5 years) without top ups or use of formula. ◆ **Naomi**

Sometimes, preemies need a special fortifier added to breastmilk for a little while. This isn't because Mum's milk is lacking, but because it helps them to grow and develop faster than without it. The fortifier is given in breastmilk, not instead of. Formula milk is widely understood to be a bad idea for most premature babies, due to the significant increase in the risk of a horrible illness called NEC (necrotizing enterocolitis).

NEC essentially kills off parts of the gastrointestinal tract, and breastmilk has been shown in studies to significantly reduce the risk of NEC developing. For example, NEC onset after Day 7 of life occurred in 15 of 443 infants (3.4%), significantly more than in the just breastmilk cohort, where NEC occurred in two of 199 infants (1%) (p=0.009) (Herrmann & Carroll, 2014).

I was told by a job that I couldn't express at work. The boss said breastfeeding is only beneficial for the first 24 hours after birth and after that, formula is just the same and therefore, she said it was pointless. ◆ **Allie**

Under UK law, it is discrimination to stop a mother expressing at work, and the courts have ruled in the mother's favour many times. I don't think we even need to discuss the statement about human milk only being beneficial for 24 hours at this point.

> *"It's impossible to get thrush on your nipples. If you are having breast pains, it has to be mastitis." Refused to even Google nipple thrush to see that it exists* ◆ **Kirsten**

Candida (thrush) grows in damp, dark environments, like a lactating breast sitting in a damp breast pad/bra/baby's mouth! 54% of women with thrush-like symptoms who were swabbed for a study were found to have thrush (Amir et al., 2013).

> *By almost everyone when I told them I would breastfeed my twins: "There is no possible way you can feed two babies when so many people don't even have enough for one!"*
>
> *My reply: "I've two boobs and two babies. I see no issue and I will make what I need."*
>
> *Me and the boys are just about to hit the 3-year mark of feeding, I've trained as a peer supporter, and now retraining as a midwife. Breastfeeding has very much changed my life!* ◆ **Katie**

I have nothing to add to Katie's sensible response. Two breasts, two babies: it is almost like nature knows what it's doing.

> *"They don't need to wake in the night. I gave all of mine a bottle of water from four weeks old if they woke; they soon stopped." I didn't even need to test that theory. Hell to the no.* ◆ **Saskia**

As we discussed in the sleep section, forcing a baby to sleep longer by overfeeding them may contribute to an increased risk of sudden infant death syndrome.

> *When seeking advice from my GP for breastfeeding support with managing thrush and nipple wounds and in serious pain, the GP informed me that stopping breastfeeding would be the best option and that my mental health was more important. She informed me that*

> *she stopped breastfeeding after a few weeks, and it was the best thing she had done. I was 8 weeks in, and I had to work so bloody hard to continue breastfeeding, and little did she know, that if I had followed her advice, it would have done the opposite she suggested, and most likely would have significantly impacted on my mental health, as I was so determined to breastfeed. I went back to get support from my IBCLC and continue to breastfeed 21 months in.* ◆ **Dionne**

There's a lot to unpack here, including the GP using her own experience (and likely triggered feelings) to try to influence someone else's feeding choices. We discuss the impact of early cessation of breastfeeding on mental health earlier on in the book, so take a look at that for more information. Essentially, as Prof. Amy Brown's work consistently shows us, making mothers stop breastfeeding *leads* to depression; it doesn't cure it.

> *Formula will settle baby better. Then, gives my 3-day-old baby a small formula top-up, as she fed non-stop but had still lost weight only to have a baby now projectile vomit and scream for four hours straight. Never did she have one again, and she is 2 years old and still breastfeeding.* ◆ **Stephanie**

Here Stephanie perfectly demonstrates that formula doesn't necessarily make life easier, like the adverts would have you believe.

> *I was told by my health visitor to eat cake every afternoon because lack of carbohydrates was causing low supply in the evenings. Also, that food with onions in it can cause reflux. Was happy to follow the first piece of advice, ignored the second.* ◆ **Becky**

I'm down for cake, but of course, there is no evidence that we need to eat more carbs to support milk supply. The onion thing is also unlikely to be true. However, some mums do report that avoiding food like onions seems to help relieve a degree of fussiness, so my suggestion is that if it's a food that you won't miss, see what happens when you avoid it. Then test your theory by eating the item in question and noticing if the fussiness returns. (Obviously, only do this if we're talking about fussiness. If you suspect a true allergy, please work with a professional to test safely.)

I'm sure this is a common one but a paediatric dietician, to whom my 12-month-old had been referred for failure to thrive, told me that breastmilk for over 1-year-olds "has no goodness in it." She also told me that I was going to have to switch to formula or cows' milk so that we could measure her intake, that her failure to gain weight could not be addressed while I was still breastfeeding due to difficulty measuring. [This is] Despite the fact that she was already on solids and taking cows' milk in a cup from time to time anyway. It seemed important to her that I stopped breastfeeding for the wellbeing of my baby. ◆ **Clover**

Sadly, when we don't know what's going on for a baby, breastfeeding tends to get the blame. It seems like it is easy to eliminate to see if there is an improvement in symptoms. This advice completely disregards the importance of breastfeeding to the nursling and parent, or whether things get worse if breastfeeding is stopped (particularly problematic when you remember how hard restarting breastfeeding can be), and the WHO guidelines for exclusive breastfeeding for 2 years and beyond.

I was told (by a midwife) that because none of the women on my husband's side of the family could breastfeed, I wouldn't be able to, despite my mother feeding three children for a relatively long time. ◆ **Frances**

This one puzzled me for a moment. My best guess is that the midwife felt that there was a problem with the babies in this family that made breastfeeding impossible. While it's possibly linked (tongue-tie tends to run in families, for example), it's the first time I have heard that the father's side would impact the mother's ability to breastfeed.

It's too hot for your baby to only have breastmilk. You need to give him water or he will dehydrate. I went on to exclusively breastfeed him through the dead of summer and he didn't suffer with dehydration once. ◆ **Alanna**

Human milk is made from close to 90% water. In hot weather, exclusively breastfed babies will usually simply feed more often, ensuring their hydration needs are well met. It can be easier for Mum to become dehydrated though, so please look after yourself while boobing.

I was told that the enormous pain I was in while feeding my new son was that my "nipples needed to toughen up." This was from a health visitor. Subsequently, [I was] told by a dental surgeon that the only reason I was having pain feeding my 1-year-old was that he had teeth and that, and I quote, I should stop breastfeeding, take him home, and give him fish and chips. ENT agreed at 18 months to divide a really thick lip and tongue-tie under a general anaesthetic. ◆ **Louise**

Another example of trust mothers here, I think.

That it's selfish to exclusively breastfeed because feeding a bottle is the "best way" to help other people bond with baby.

Is it not selfish of that person to expect to be entitled to bond with your baby through their choice of feeding, instead of just holding them and talking to them?

Let's be honest, feeding a bottle is time consuming, takes two hands, and is just a bit boring. [You] Have to stare at them to make sure they're not drowning or choking and can't even reach for a biscuit! ◆ **Abbey**

This quote is a favourite of mine, not the least because Abbey's rage is on point.

My funniest was when a new mum was told that if her baby fell asleep on the breast, it would blow air back into her breasts. Can you imagine all those inflated boobs? ◆ **Rayanne**

At this point, I have no sensible commentary to add. I mean, that's not how any of this works.

There are over 500 other quotes in a post on my Facebook page at the time of writing, but I just don't have the room to include them all. I think these parents have summed up the other chapters in this book perfectly; there is a lot of nonsense out there about breastfeeding, and it is still being spread widely in 2021.

CHAPTER 14

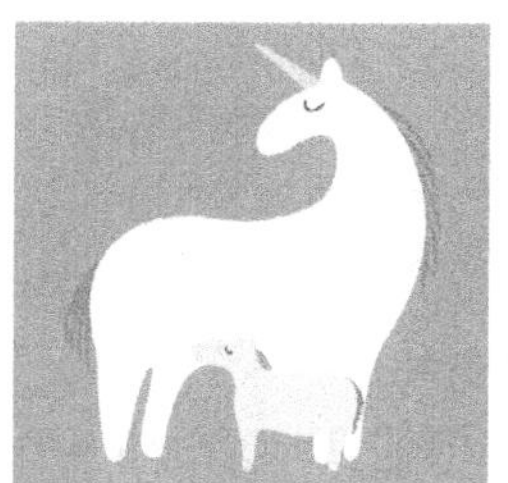

Final Thoughts and Seeking More Help

This book has not been the most enjoyable one to write. The sheer level of misinformation floating around about breastfeeding is depressing, particularly because most of it is easily disproved nonsense. While what we read and are told usually is well-intentioned, it damages breastfeeding relationships. Most of the myths in this book have an undertone of misogyny and distrust of women's bodies. A lot of the poor advice centres around "you can't do X," where "you" refers to the lactating parent. Breastfeeding seems to magnify the already huge gap between men and women in a Western, patriarchal society with a clear message that it is weird, vaguely sexual, and there's no way you can feed this child.

The fact that we are told, instead, to feed our babies milk from a lactating cow is an irony that continues to puzzle me. Dairy cows are given extra food, rest, and all sorts of tests when their milk yield is down, but a woman is just told to get some powdered milk off a shelf. Of course, there is a whole other argument here about the dairy industry, which also profits off of human babies not getting human milk, but it's not one I have the space to get into here.

During the years I have worked and volunteered in breastfeeding support, I've become convinced that reaching your breastfeeding goal is a big two fingers up to our culture, the patriarchy, and misogynists everywhere. Unfortunately, most breastfeeding parents will, at some point or another, come across damaging information (often unsolicited). It takes balls to ignore that and keep going with what you believe is right. Women have been threatened with children's services on a fairly regular basis for refusing to give formula, wanting to give donor milk acquired by a peer, or breastfeeding for "too long" among a list of other bizarre reasons. When did feeding our babies and children according to our biological and evolutionary norm become controversial while feeding them milk from another species has become the accepted norm?

On the other hand, bottle-feeding is normalised. You are told to breastfeed until that baby is born and you run into problems. Then, the clock is ticking before someone mentions formula, blames a lack of milk, or declares that Fed is Best. Mothers cannot win. They breastfeed and they are criticised, given bad information, and are not supported. They don't breastfeed and they get the same treatment.

Approximately 80% of women want to breastfeed, but 80% of them also say they stopped before they were ready. Researching this book brought home exactly why that is. It seems impossible to just get on with feeding your baby. Support we need and deserve is, at best, patchy. At worst, it's offered by people with lanyards, white coats, or the matriarch of a family, with absolutely no regard to what the mother wants. The message is clear: we can't trust mothers to know what they are doing, and we can't trust their strange female bodies to produce the milk required to grow another human. After all, if she succeeds, no one will make a profit off her.

Speaking of profits, many issues we see are fuelled by the poor ethics of formula companies. Your money is worth a lot to them. If they can get you using their formula, you will be a loyal customer for at least 12 months. Their appalling practices, proven to harm babies and mothers the world over, put profit above health. Remember, formula is not the problem; formula marketing is. There is an important distinction, and blaming mums who are backed into a formula-feeding corner by the sort of misinformation we have seen in this book doesn't help anyone.

Safeguarding Your Breastfeeding Goals

So, if you're breastfeeding, how do you safeguard your breastfeeding relationship and smash your goals?

1. Read books like this, and if necessary, use the citations to back up what you are saying when people challenge me. It annoys me hugely that this is something I have to suggest, because a mother's choices should be accepted without the need for scientific evidence. However, we know that isn't the case, so backing up your right to breastfeed in a certain situation with a published paper will usually silence most well-meaning people.

2. Ask anyone questioning you for the evidence to back up their claim, especially if it's a health professional. If you are in a medical setting, ask to see the policy that states what you have been told. They usually can't produce either.

3. When you have a breastfeeding problem, seek skilled help from a helpline, breastfeeding champion, support worker, midwife, health visitor, peer supporter, breastfeeding counsellor, or an IBCLC or infant feeding lead.

4. If what you are told is not correct, get another opinion. Yes, even if the opinion is from someone you usually trust. If it seems a bit off, ask someone else. Also ask for the research that backs up what they're telling you. Even the best make mistakes or have gaps in their knowledge.

5. Be an advocate. Speak up and correct people when you know they're wrong. Breastfeed your nursling in public, talk about it, take photos, and share articles. Be the One Who Breastfeeds to your friends, family, and work colleagues. They will come to you when they have problems. You might even consider training to be a peer supporter or breastfeeding counsellor!

Together, we can change the world for our children so they can breastfeed without all the stresses, strains, and arguments we went through.

Acknowledgements

As always, books don't come together on their own. Numerous people are involved both directly and indirectly. I'd like to start by thanking my social media community for always being so open when it comes to sharing their experiences. You can see many of their quotes throughout this book, and this is because I firmly believe that their voices need to be heard. What parents are experiencing is real, and they have kindly shared those experiences with us in these pages.

I'd also like to thank The Queer Parenting Partnership. Kim looked over my information for trans and nonbinary folk, gave me some things to think about, and checked that I was being the best ally possible for that section.

Jessie Cuming, Sarah Oakley, and Sian Aldis, for casting their experienced eyes over my final draft to ensure my information was evidence-based.

Ken Tackett and Kathleen Kendall-Tackett at Praeclarus Press for always being patient with my inability to meet deadlines or to use the correct format for my references.

Charlotte Bond. This is the third book she has edited for me now, and I am convinced she is the reason people buy my work. She takes the ramblings of an ADHD brain and turns them into concise, sensibly structured sentences.

On a personal note, 2021 has been a hard year for me. I would like to thank my friends and family, who have never wavered in their support, both practical and emotional, even when I was, frankly, a puddle.

I should also thank the Premier Inn in Poole, Dorset because that is where most of this book was written over 3 days, 2 weeks before my editing deadline, fuelled by their coffee and the bliss of no laundry or dishes to contend with, and no one interrupting me to demand snacks.

References

Alaluusua, S., Myllarniemi, S., Kallio, M., Salmenpera, L., & Tainio, V. (1990). Prevalence of caries and salivary levels of mutans streptococci in 5-year-old children in relation to duration of breast feeding. *European Journal of Oral Sciences, 98*(3), 193-196. *doi: 10.1111/j.1600-0722.1990.tb00961.x*

Alsaweed, M. et al. (2016). Human milk cells and lipids conserve numerous known and novel miRNAs, some of which are differentially expressed during lactation. *PLoS One, 11*(4):e0152610.

Amir, L., Donath, S., Garland, S., Tabrizi, S., Bennett, C., Cullinane, M., & Payne, M. (2013). DoesCandidaand/orStaphylococcusplay a role in nipple and breast pain in lactation? A cohort study in Melbourne, Australia. *BMJ Open, 3*(3), e002351. doi: 10.1136/bmjopen-2012-002351

Anstey, E. H., Shoemaker, M. L., Barrera, C. M., O'Neil, M. E., Verma, A. B., & Holman, D. M. (2017). Breastfeeding and breast cancer risk reduction: Implications for black mothers. *American Journal of Preventive Medicine, 53*(3S1), S40–S46. https://doi.org/10.1016/j.amepre.2017.04.024

Anttila-Huges, J. K., Fernald, L.C. H., Gertler, P.G., Krause, P., & Wydick, B. (2018). Mortality from Nestle's marketing of infant formula in low and middle-income countries. *Working Paper 24452* http://www.nber.org/papers/w24452

Avery, M. D., Duckett, L., & Frantzich, C. R. (2000). The experience of sexuality during breastfeeding among primiparous women. *Journal of Midwifery & Women's Health, 45*(3), 227–237. https://doi.org/10.1016/s1526-9523(00)00020-9

Ballard, O., & Morrow, A. (2013). Human milk composition: Nutrients and bioactive factors. *Pediatric Clinics of North America, 60*(1), 49-74.

BASIS online. (n.d.). *The costs of sleep training.* https://www.basisonline.org.uk/hcp-the-costs-of-sleep-training/).

Bugental, D. B., Martorell, G. A., & Barraza, V. (2003). The hormonal costs of subtle forms of infant maltreatment. *Hormones & Behavior, 43*(1), 237-44. doi: 10.1016/s0018-506x(02)00008-9. PMID: 12614655.

Brown, A., Rance, J., & Bennett, P. (2015). Understanding the relationship between breastfeeding and postnatal depression: The role of pain and physical difficulties. *Journal of Advanced Nursing, 72*(2), 273-282. doi: 10.1111/jan.12832

Chen, E., Gau, M., Liu, C., & Lee, T. (2017). Effects of father-neonate skin-to-skin contact on attachment: A randomized controlled trial. *Nursing Research and Practice, 2017, 1-8. doi: 10.1155/2017/8612024*

Clemons, S.N., & Amir, L.H. (2010). Breastfeeding women's experience of expressing: A descriptive study. *Journal of Human Lactation. 26*(3), 258-265. doi:10.1177/0890334410371209

Cowie, J., Holland, P., Pirie, I., & Milligan, C. (2018). Patterns of prescribing in the management of gastro-oesophageal reflux in infants in Scotland. *Journal of Health Visiting, 6*(9), 440-446. doi: 10.12968/johv.2018.6.9.440

Davis, M. K. (1998). Review of the evidence for an association between infant feeding and childhood cancer. *International Journal of Cancer, 11*, 29-33.

Dieterich, C., Felice, J., O'Sullivan, E., & Rasmussen, K. (2013). Breastfeeding and health outcomes for the mother-infant dyad. *Pediatric Clinics of North America, 60*(1), 31-48. doi: 10.1016/j.pcl.2012.09.010

Doan, T., Gardiner, A., Gay, C. L., & Lee, K. A. (2007). Breast-feeding increases sleep duration of new parents. *The Journal of Perinatal & Neonatal Nursing, 21*(3), 200–206. https://doi.org/10.1097/01.JPN.0000285809.36398.1b

Dorheim, S.K., Bondevik, G.T., Eberhard-Gran, M., & Bjorvatn, B. (2009). Sleep and depression in postpartum women: A population-based study. *Sleep, 32*(7), 847-855.

Doucet, S., Soussignan, R., Sagot, P., & Schaal, B. (2009). The secretion of areolar (Montgomery's) glands from lactating women elicits selective, unconditional responses in neonates. *Plos ONE, 4*(10), e7579. doi: 10.1371/journal.pone.0007579.

Drugs and Lactation Database (LactMed). (2020). *Alcohol.* Bethesda (MD): National Library of Medicine (US). https://www.ncbi.nlm.nih.gov/books/NBK501469/

Duncan, B., Ey, J., Holberg, C. J., Wright, A. L., Martinez, F. D., & Taussig, L. M. (1993). Exclusive breast-feeding for at least 4 months protects against otitis media. *Pediatrics, 91*(5), 867–872.

Elias, M., & Nicolson, N. & Bora, C., & Johnston, J. (1986). Sleep/wake patterns of breast-fed infants in the first 2 years of life. *Pediatrics, 77*, 322-329.

Erickson, P.R., & Mazhari, E. (1999). Investigation of the role of human breast milk in caries development. *Pediatric Den*tistry *21*(2), 86-90.

Evans, K. (2003). Effect of caesarean section on breast milk transfer to the normal term newborn over the first week of life. *Archives of Disease in Childhood - Fetal and Neonatal Edition, 88*(5), 380F-382. doi: 10.1136/fn.88.5.f380

Fabic, M., & Choi, Y. (2013). Assessing the quality of data regarding use of the lactational amenorrhea method. *Studies in Family Planning, 44*(2), 205-221. doi: 10.1111/j.1728-4465.2013.00353.x

Flower, H. (2003). *Adventures in tandem nursing: Breastfeeding during pregnancy and beyond.* La Leche League International.

Ford, B., Lam, P., John, O., & Mauss, I. (2018). The psychological health benefits of accepting negative emotions and thoughts: Laboratory, diary, and longitudinal evidence. *Journal of Personality and Social Psychology, 115*(6), 1075-1092.

Haham, A., Marom, R., Mangel, L., Botzer, E., & Dollberg, S. (2014). Prevalence of breastfeeding difficulties in newborns with a lingual frenulum: A prospective cohort series.*Breastfeeding Medicine*, 9(9), 438-441.

Herrmann, K., & Carroll, K. (2014). An exclusively human milk diet reduces necrotizing enterocolitis. *Breastfeeding Medicine* 9(4), 184–190. https://doi.org/10.1089/bfm.2013.0121

Horwood, L., & Fergusson, D. (1998). Breastfeeding and later cognitive and academic outcomes. *Pediatrics, 101*(1), e9-e9.

Howie, P. W., Forsyth, J. S., Ogston, S. A., Clark, A., & Florey, C. D. (1990). Protective effect of breast feeding against infection. *BMJ* (Clinical research ed.), *300*(6716), 11–16. https://doi.org/10.1136/bmj.300.6716.11

Huffman, S., Chowdhury, A., Allen, H., & Nahar, L. (1987). Suckling patterns and post-partum amenorrhoea in Bangladesh. *Journal of Biosocial Science, 19*(2), 171-179. doi:10.1017/S0021932000016771

İsik, Y., Dag, Z., Tulmac, O., & Pek, E. (2016). Early postpartum lactation effects of cesarean and vaginal birth. *Ginekologia Polska, 87(6), 426-430.*

Joas, J., Mohler, E. (2021) Maternal bonding in early infancy predicts childrens' social competences in preschool age. *Frontiers in Psychiatry, 12*.doi 10.3389/fpsyt.2021.687535

Jones, W. (2021). *Factsheet on codeine*. Breastfeeding Network. https://www.breastfeedingnetwork.org.uk/codeine/).

Kendall-Tackett, K.A., Cong, Z., Hale, T.W. (2011). The effect of feeding method on sleep duration, maternal well-being, and postpartum depression. *Clinical Lactation,* 2(2), 22-26.

Kent, J., Mitoulas, L., Cregan, M., Ramsay, D., Doherty, D., & Hartmann, P. (2006). Volume and frequency of breastfeedings and fat content of breast milk throughout the day. *Pediatrics, 117*(3), e387-e395.

Kent, J., Geddes, D., Hepworth, A., & Hartmann, P. (2011). Effect of warm breastshields on breast milk pumping. *Journal of Human Lactation*, *27*(4), 331-338.

Krol, K. M., & Grossmann, T. (2018). Psychological effects of breastfeeding on children and mothers. [Psychologische effekte des stillens auf kinder und mütter. bundesgesundheitsblatt, gesundheitsforschung], *Gesundheitsschutz, 61*(8), 977–985. https://doi.org/10.1007/s00103-018-2769-0

Lagercrantz, H., & Changeux, J. (2009). The emergence of human consciousness: From fetal to neonatal life. *Pediatric Research, 65*(3),.255-260.

Leonard, L.G. (2000). Breastfeeding triplets: The at-home experience. *Public Health Nursing, 17,* 211-221. https://doi.org/10.1046/j.1525-1446.2000.00211.x

Little, E., Legare, C., & Carver, L. (2018). Mother–infant physical contact predicts responsive feeding among U.S. breastfeeding mothers. *Nutrients, 10*(9), 1251.

Maher, V. (Ed.). (1992). *Anthropology of breast-feeding: Natural law or social construct* (Vol. 3). Berg Publishers.

Mead, L., Chuffo, R., Lawlor-Klean, P., & Meier, P. (1992). Breastfeeding success with preterm quadruplets. *Journal of Obstetric, Gynecologic, & Neonatal Nursing, 21*(3), 221-227.

Mohrbacher, N. (2010). *Breastfeeding answers made simple*. Hale Publications

Morton, J. (2017). *Maximizing milk production with hands-on pumping.* https://med.stanford.edu/newborns/professional-education/breastfeeding/maximizing-milk-production.html

Mueller, L. S. J. (1985). Pregnancy and sexuality. *Journal of Obstetric, Gynecologic, & Neonatal Nursing, 14*(4), 289-294.

National Institute for Health Care and Excellence (NICE). (2019). *Gastro-oesophageal reflux disease in children and young people: Diagnosis and management*. https://www.ncbi.nlm.nih.gov/books/NBK552673/

Oakley, S. (2021). *Why tongue-tie matters*. Pinter & Martin.

Patnaik, S., Sharma, S., Sinha, S., & Roy, K. (1999). Case study of a lactating grandmother. *Indian Journal of Public Health, 43*(1), 10, 25. PMID: 11243080.

Simon, A., Hollander, G., & McMichael, A. (2015). Evolution of the immune system in humans from infancy to old age. *Proceedings of the Royal Society B: Biological Sciences*, 282(1821), 20143085.

Sinkiewicz-Darol, E., Bernatowicz-Łojko, U., Łubiech, K., Adamczyk, I., Twarużek, M., Baranowska, B., Skowron, K., & Spatz, D., 2021. Tandem breastfeeding: A descriptive analysis of the nutritional value of milk when feeding a younger and older child. *Nutrients, 13*(1), 277.

Santoro, W., Jr, Martinez, F. E., Ricco, R. G., & Jorge, S. M. (2010). *Colostrum ingested during the first day of life by exclusively breastfed healthy newborn infants.* The Journal of pediatrics, 156(1), 29–32. https://doi.org/10.1016/j.jpeds.2009.07.009

Sugimura, T., Seo, T., Terasaki, N., Ozaki, Y., Rikitake, N., Okabe, R., & Matsushita, M. (2021).Efficacy and safety of breast milk eye drops in infants with eye discharge. *ActaPaediatrics, 110,* 1322-1329. https://doi.org/10.1111/apa.15628

Thompson, J., Tanabe, K., Moon, R., Mitchell, E., McGarvey, C., Tappin, D., Blair, P., & Hauck, F. (2017). Duration of breastfeeding and risk of SIDS: An individual participant data meta-analysis. *Pediatrics, 140*(5), e20171324

Townsend, J. A., Brannon, R. B., Cheramie, T., & Hagan, J. (2014). Prevalence and variations of the median maxillary labial frenum in children, adolescents, and adults in a diverse population. *General Dentistry, 61*(2), 57-60; quiz 61. PMID: 23454324.

Wilson, A. C., Forsyth, J. S., Greene, S. A., Irvine, L., Hau, C., & Howie, P. W. (1998). Relation of infant diet to childhood health: seven year follow up of cohort of children in Dundee infant feeding study. *BMJ (Clinical research ed.), 316*(7124), 21–25. https://doi.org/10.1136/bmj.316.7124.21

Wood, K., & van Esterik, P. (2011). Infant feeding experiences of women who were sexually abused in childhood. *Canadian Family Physician. 56*(4), e136-e141.

Zhou, L., Yoshimura, Y., Huang, Y., Suzuki, R., Yokoyama, M., Okabe, M., & Shimamura, M., (2000). Two independent pathways of maternal cell transmission to offspring: Through placenta during pregnancy and by breast-feeding after birth. *Immunology, 101*(4), 570-580.

Made in the USA
Middletown, DE
23 November 2022

15672423R00106